EFFECTIVE ANGER MANAGEMENT

FOR CHILDREN AND YOUTH

The Manual

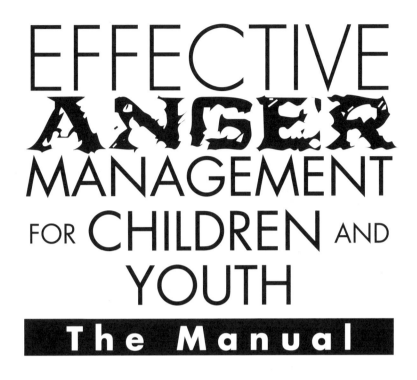

EFFECTIVE ANGER MANAGEMENT FOR CHILDREN AND YOUTH
The Manual

Yoon Phaik Ooi
University of Basel, Switzerland

Rebecca P. Ang
Nanyang Technological University, Singapore

Nikki Lim-Ashworth
Institute of Mental Health, Singapore

Illustrated by Yan Lin Tan

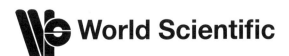

World Scientific

NEW JERSEY • LONDON • SINGAPORE • BEIJING • SHANGHAI • HONG KONG • TAIPEI • CHENNAI

Published by

World Scientific Publishing Co. Pte. Ltd.

5 Toh Tuck Link, Singapore 596224

USA office: 27 Warren Street, Suite 401-402, Hackensack, NJ 07601

UK office: 57 Shelton Street, Covent Garden, London WC2H 9HE

Library of Congress Cataloging-in-Publication Data
Ooi, Yoon Phaik, author.
   Effective anger management for children and youth : the manual and the workbook / by Yoon Phaik Ooi,
Rebecca P. Ang, Nikki Lim-Ashworth.
      p. ; cm.
   Includes bibliographical references and index.
   ISBN 978-9814596121 (pbk. : alk. paper)
   I. Ang, Rebecca P., author. II. Lim-Ashworth, Nikki, author. III. Title.
   [DNLM: 1. Anger--Programmed Instruction. 2. Adolescent. 3. Aggression--Programmed Instruction. 4. Child.
5. Cognitive Therapy--methods--Programmed Instruction. WS 18.2]
   RJ506.A35
   155.4'1247--dc23
                                    2014001210

British Library Cataloguing-in-Publication Data
A catalogue record for this book is available from the British Library.

Printed in Singapore

About the Authors

Yoon Phaik Ooi, Ph.D., is a Research Scientist with the Division of Clinical Psychology and Psychotherapy, Department of Psychology, University of Basel, Switzerland. She is also an Adjunct Assistant Professor with the DUKE-NUS Graduate Medical School, Singapore and Visiting Research Fellow with the Department of Child and Adolescent Psychiatry, Institute of Mental Health, Singapore. She is an independent trainer of the Autism Diagnostic Interview–Revised (ADI-R). Her research interests include developmental psychopathology and intervention work with children and adolescents at risk for behavioural and emotional problems such as Disruptive Behaviour Disorders and Autism Spectrum Disorders. She is actively involved in research and has published widely in the area of child and adolescent mental health.

Rebecca P. Ang, Ph.D., is an Associate Professor at Psychological Studies Academic Group, National Institute of Education, Nanyang Technological University, Singapore. She is a Nationally Certified School Psychologist in the USA, and a Registered Psychologist in Singapore. Her research and professional interests include developmental child psychopathology and, in particular, antisocial and aggressive behavior, and related prevention and intervention work. She is also interested in parent–child relationships, teacher–student relationships, and the impact of the quality of such relationships on child, familial and school adjustment and functioning.

Ms. Nikki Lim-Ashworth has been a Psychologist with the Department of Child and Adolescent Psychiatry, Institute of Mental Health, Singapore, since 2008. She received her M.A. in Applied Psychology from the National Institute of Education, Nanyang Technological University, Singapore. She is currently pursuing her Doctorate in Clinical Psychology with the University

College London, UK. She is involved in several research studies on disruptive behaviour disorders. Her other research interest includes the role of emotional regulation in childhood anxiety. She facilitates specialised parenting programmes for parents with children with ADHD and individualised cognitive behavioural therapy for children with mood and anxiety concerns.

Acknowledgements

The authors would like to thank Caroline, Delia, Jean, Jen, Liying, Xinyi, and Yan Lin from the SASSI team for their help in facilitating the social problem-solving skills groups conducted at the Child Guidance Clinic. They gratefully acknowledge their inputs and ideas in their work through the numerous discussions they have had about these group sessions.

This book is linked to a mobile app game, called RegnaTales, which can be found at www.regnatales.com

Contents

Introduction

Problem-solving and social skills are essential life skills for children to become socially responsible adults. It is vital that young people learn to manage and regulate their emotions, communicate with each other effectively and possess positive coping strategies to handle conflict successfully. Some children seem to be constantly angry — they struggle with behavioural difficulties as demonstrated by defiance, fighting, cursing and name-calling. The strategies and activities presented in this manual and workbook will be particularly helpful for children with behavioural problems. Throughout the manual, the term 'children' will be used to refer to *both* children and adolescents.

This resource manual is specially designed for teachers, counselors, social workers, psychologists and other mental health professionals who assist in various capacities in working with children who exhibit such problems. The ideas, materials, suggested activities and games included in this resource book are applicable to both primary and secondary school children. The purpose of this resource book is to provide practical strategies divided into 12 lessons that teachers and mental health professionals can implement; it is a "how-to" book on enhancing children's problem-solving and social skills. Teachers and mental health professionals should exercise flexibility when using this manual and workbook — some may find it helpful to adapt these materials to suit the specific children they are working with (either to simplify it further for the children in Primary 1 and 2 or to elaborate on certain skills and concepts to make it more meaningful and relevant for the adolescents in Secondary 4).

Through these 12 lessons, children are taught a variety of positive coping techniques for problem-solving, conflict management as well as anger control. As children's problem behaviours decrease and their positive coping resources increase, they will gain a more positive attitude towards school and the schooling process. This in turn will contribute towards their academic, social and emotional enhancement.

- **Format:** These lessons can be delivered to children individually or in a small group of between four to eight children of similar age and development. It can also be used with a class of 40 pupils. The book is written as if these lessons are to be taught to a group of children, but these lessons can also be taught to children individually.

- **Facilitators:** Facilitators can include teachers, teacher-counsellors, counsellors, social workers, psychologists and other mental health professionals.

- **Setting:** The structure of the lessons is designed to accommodate participants from a variety of settings including schools, family service centres, and community rehabilitation facilities.

- **Facilities:** Minimal facilities are required. A classroom, conference room or counselling room should suffice.

- **Duration:** 12 lessons in total. Each lesson lasts for approximately 45 minutes to 60 minutes. Depending on the setting, lessons may be conducted once a week, twice weekly or fortnightly. Facilitators have the flexibility to lengthen the lessons to 90 minutes if further discussion is needed. Facilitators can also use an extra lesson or two to teach the content of a particular session if they feel that children they are working with are in need of extra coaching in that area.

The content of these 12 lessons specifically target the various cognitive-behavioural difficulties manifested by children with anger or behavioural problems. These children have difficulty in identifying feelings accurately. They selectively attend to and recall aggressive cues, almost to the exclusion of other non-aggressive cues making them misperceive many social situations, hence leading to potential fights and misunderstandings.

Lesson 1 focuses on the identification of feelings in children and begins with children identifying and discussing a wide range of feelings including pleasant (e.g., calm, joyful and hopeful) and unpleasant (e.g., sad, angry, lonely and guilty) feelings they have experienced. Children are taught to identify clues that could help them to understand feelings such as words (what people say), tone of voice, body language and the situation. Lesson 2 targets and teaches specifically feelings underlying anger and associated with anger. It teaches strategies to help children recognise anger triggers in their physical bodies (e.g., feeling tensed or relaxed), thoughts (e.g., I want to hit him) and actions (e.g., punch). Children are taught to understand that anger feelings can range from mild (e.g., irritable), to moderate (e.g., frustrated) or severe (e.g., enraged), and help them articulate what makes them angry or calm. Following that, children are guided to understand the distinction between feelings and behaviour, and that feelings influence but do not dictate their behaviours. While children are taught to normalise and accept their angry feelings, they are also reminded the three Anger Rules: (1) it is not okay to hurt myself when I am angry; (2) it is not okay to hurt/hit others (including animals) when I am angry; and (3) it is not okay to destroy things when I am angry.

Lessons 3 and 4 are designed to teach children various anger-coping techniques such as deep breathing, visualisation, muscle relaxation, leisure activities, positive self-talk, asking for help and assertive management of intense emotions and difficult situations. The therapist can choose to teach three to four anger-coping techniques that are most appropriate for their group of children. In these lessons, children are asked to identify situations that typically arouse their intense, angry feelings and practise anger-coping strategies to inhibit automatic and impulsive responses. Children are encouraged to use these anger-coping techniques when they encounter angry situations as part of their homework. Lessons 5 and 6 are structured to teach children empathy and perspective-taking skills. Through these lessons and activities, children are guided to recognise other people's feelings (empathy), see things from other people's point of view and pay attention to social cues inconsistent with attribution of hostile intent (perspective-taking). To practise empathy skills, children will participate in a discussion of social encounters that involve identifying other people's feelings and the impact of their behaviours towards them. To practise perspective-taking skills, children will participate in a discussion of social encounters that involve discriminating between accidental and intentional actions, and share experiences and reactions to hypothetical situations. This enables the child to gradually recognise the possibility that negative social encounters could be the result of an accident and may not always be intentional.

Lesson 7 focuses on Fighting Fair, another method of resolving frustration and conflict by building rather than tearing down relationships, and it allows anger to be expressed in a healthy way (Shapiro & Cole, 1994). In Fighting Fair, children are taught five rules: (1) attack the problem, not the person; (2) listen to the other person and allow for disagreement; (3) respect the other person's feelings; (4) take responsibility for your own actions; and (5) avoid 'fouls'. Children apply this strategy to simple hypothetical problem situations and to real-life problems. They practise using verbal mediation or "self-talk" (Meichenbaum, 1977) as a strategy to remind them to control impulses, think about consequences of actions and reinforce their own behaviours. Lesson 8 teaches children prosocial skills such as sharing, cooperation, helping, making friends and keeping out of fights. Many children who display behavioural difficulties have developed such a repertoire of unacceptable behaviours over many years such that these negative behaviours become almost part of these children's personality and self-image. The homework exercise based on 'Random Acts of Kindness' helps to gradually reverse this negative downward spiral by deliberately putting children in situations where they will behave well and even in altruistic ways.

Lessons 9 to 11 focus on teaching children effective problem-solving methods. The five-step problem-solving strategy (also known as the ANGER Plan) addresses each of the processes from the social information processing model that contributes to socially competent behaviour such as accurate encoding and interpretation of relevant social cues, generation and evaluation of potential responses, and behavioural enactment of a selected response (Crick & Dodge, 1994). Children are taught the following steps:

(1) Feeling Angry? (2) Do Not React First; (3) Generate Solutions; (4) Evaluation Solutions; and (5) Reflect and Reward. Table 2 presents further details of the ANGER Plan.

Lesson 12 serves as the summary and integrative review session. This lesson requires children to demonstrate what they have learnt from previous lessons. It would also be an appropriate time for the facilitator to empower the children to continue to maintain the coping skills they have acquired even after the 12 lessons have been completed.

Session 1: Identification of Feelings in Ourselves and Others

> *Overview of Activities:*
>
> 1. Introduction to group — establish rules and reward system
> 2. Warm-up activity
> 3. Identification of feelings
> 4. Summary

1. *WELCOME* each member to the group.

2. *INTRODUCE* the facilitator to the group. Learn each others' names.

3. *WARM-UP ACTIVITY*. BINGO Friendship game (see Friendship Bingo template in Appendix 1).

4. *INTRODUCTION TO SOCIAL PROBLEM-SOLVING SKILLS TRAINING*. Tell the group that they are here to learn some skills that would be useful for them.

5. Establish *RULES* and expectations for the group. Allow the group to brainstorm ideas about rules and expectations.

6. Establish *REWARD SYSTEM* for the group.

7. *IDENTIFICATION OF FEELINGS*. Facilitate the discussion on various feelings of human emotions. Guide the group to identify various feelings in themselves and others. Get the group to role-play these feelings while sharing their experiences.

8. *CONCLUSION*. Conclude the meeting with a summary of what the group has learnt about the identification of various feelings in themselves and in others. Encourage children to attempt the worksheets as part of their homework.

Session 1
Identification of Feelings in Ourselves and Others

1. *Introduction and Rationale*

   ▪ Essential to learn the names of the children in the group.

   ▪ Learn about the wide range of feelings in ourselves and in others.

   ▪ Learn how to cope with angry feelings and how to express them in acceptable ways.

   ▪ Learn good ways of solving problems.

   ▪ Learn how to resolve conflict without resorting to hitting, shouting and threatening.

   ▪ These skills will be learnt through games, role-playing, activities and discussions.

2. *Establish Rules and Determine Reward System*

   ▪ Establish rules and expectations for the group.

   ▪ Have group members brainstorm ideas about rules and expectations for the group.

   ▪ Discuss and process with group members regarding the purpose of these rules. These rules are present for the smooth functioning of the group so that all group members can benefit from the group learning experience and enjoy the activities.

   ▪ Examples of some useful rules include the following: a) respect others (e.g., no teasing, no put-downs and respect other people's personal space); b) use appropriate language (e.g., no swearing); c) attend meetings regularly;

d) be productive and participate actively within the group; e) be punctual for meetings; and f) complete homework.

- If this programme is implemented as part of a Civics and Moral Education lesson in class, then regular classroom rules will apply. If facilitators are working with individual children, appropriate rules and expectations can be worked out between the child and the facilitator.

- These rules and expectations can be written and posted on a large vanguard sheet for use in subsequent skills training sessions.

- The facilitator will need to determine the following: type of reward/incentive, frequency and condition attached to the distribution of these incentives. Type of reward may be in the form of candy, pencils or pens. Frequency refers to how often you wish to provide the reward for group members. The facilitator may decide to provide the incentive on a weekly or fortnightly basis, or he/she may decide to provide rewards on a random basis. Condition refers to the elements that need to be present before a particular incentive or reward is provided. For example, the facilitator may decide that group participation and adherence to group rules/expectations are necessary preconditions for the distribution of the reward/incentive.

3. *Warm-up Activity*

- The facilitator may choose to play Friendship Bingo (Appendix 1) or to come up with another suitable activity for group members to get to know one another better. Friendship Bingo is an activity for children to be more familiar with one another prior to the commencement of the group. Each child participating in the activity needs to have a copy of the Friendship Bingo activity sheet. In this activity, children approach other participants to sign the appropriate square on their Friendship Bingo sheet if the participant fits that particular description (e.g., "Is the youngest in the family"). The winner is the first person to complete collecting signatures for an entire row, column or diagonal. The difficulty level of this activity can be adjusted depending on the number of participants one has in the group. The difficulty level of Friendship Bingo can be increased (depending on the number of people participating in the group) by having the facilitator place a couple of restrictions on the game. For example, the facilitator could state that the number of signatures that the child can obtain from the same person is limited to five (or less), and in order to win the game, five signatures obtained from the same person cannot be found on an entire row, column or diagonal.

4. *Identification of Feelings*

■   The objective of this segment is for group members to demonstrate knowledge of a wide range of possible human emotions and to identify these emotions in others. Children need to better understand the relationship between their feelings and their behaviour, and the first step towards this understanding is to consider the wide range of emotions that humans are capable of. The foundation of emotional well-being is the ability to understand and express one's own feelings appropriately. For aggressive children, the feeling of anger is often so salient that underlying feelings such as hurt, rejection, anxiety, embarrassment and the like are often obscured. Becoming aware of these other feelings facilitates effective problem-solving (Dodge, Laird, Lochman, Zelli, & Conduct Problems Prevention Research Group, 2002; Kusche & Greenberg, 1994; Mostow, Izard, Fine, & Trentacosta, 2002).

■   The group facilitator can decide on the best way to implement this segment of the session based on the age, developmental level and composition of the group members. The "Feelings Word Bank" worksheet can be used as a guide to increase children's vocabulary and understanding of feelings words. For younger children, the facilitator might want to choose five feelings words to focus on instead of the entire list. Generate group discussion on different situations that might create certain feelings. Actively involve the children in discussing situations that might bring about different feelings. While doing so, help children understand that it is normal to experience pleasant and unpleasant feelings.

■ The facilitator can teach children to look for clues that identify a person's feelings such as the look on a person's face (i.e., facial expression), words, tone of voice, body language and the situation the person is experiencing. Teaching children to look out for such clues may increase their ability to be attuned to the feelings of others.

■ The facilitator can have group members participate in one or more of the following suggested activities:

a) **Feelings-Charade.** The children could play Feelings-Charade using the 45 feelings cards provided in Appendix 2. Feelings-Charade is a game that helps children identify the important non-verbal cues (gestures, actions and facial expressions) that reveal emotions. These feelings cards can be detached by cutting along the dotted lines. Divide the children into two or more groups depending on the total number of participants present. **Variation 1:** Each child draws a feeling card and acts out the feelings stated on the card while team members attempt to guess the feeling portrayed. The facilitator can pre-select a sample of feelings cards to be used or he/she can choose to play Feelings Charade using all the cards. **Variation 2:** Have the children sit together in a circle. Each child draws a feeling card (without looking at it) and attaches it onto their foreheads. The other children provide clues for the child to guess the feeling word on his or her forehead. The children are not allowed to verbalise the feeling word directly but can provide cues such as tone of voice, describe a situation where the feeling is associated, demonstrate behaviour cues of the feelings, etc.

b) **Feelings-Word.** The objective of this Feelings-Word game is for team members to guess the "feelings word" with the child providing only verbal clues. The "Feelings Word Bank" provided (see Appendix 3) can be used as the list of feelings words. For example, the word is 'nervous'. The child can provide verbal clues such as "I feel this way just before an exam", "I feel this way if I have to give a speech in front of the whole school during morning assembly" and "When I feel this way, my palms feel sweaty and my heart beats fast". Once again, the facilitator can choose to use all the cards or pre-select a sample of cards to be used.

c) **Feelings-Pictionary.** The objective of this game is for the child to draw clues so that team mates can guess the "feelings word". Once again, the feelings cards provided can be used for playing Feelings-Pictionary.

d) **Feelings-Mask.** The purpose of this activity is to help the child look at the differences between how he/she feels inside and how he/she acts on the outside. The facilitator would need to provide the child with two paper plates, one ice-cream stick, marker pens and a stapler. On one plate, ask the child to draw how he/she feels most of the time on the inside, and on the other, ask the child to draw how others see him/her on the outside. Tell the child to place the ice-cream stick between the two plates before putting them together. Actively involve the children in discussing situations that might bring about different feelings.

■ Help children understand that feelings can range from mild to moderate or severe. Use the "Feelings Meter" (see Figure 1) as a visual aid to help the child chart what makes him/her feel the different levels and intensities of feelings. The facilitator can help the child articulate the people places or things that make him/

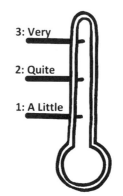

3: Very

2: Quite

1: A Little

Figure 1.   Feelings Mater

her this way. For example, certain situations can make the child feel mildly happy and other situations can make the child feel extremely happy.

5. *Summary*

- The facilitator concludes the session with a summary of what the children learnt regarding the identification of a wide range of emotions in themselves and in others.

- Homework:

   a) **Sorting out pleasant and unpleasant feelings.** Children can sort out the list of feeling words provided into pleasant and unpleasant categories (see worksheet on "Pleasant and Unpleasant Feelings").

   b) **Identification of Feelings.** Encourage children to practice identifying their own feelings as part of their homework (see worksheet on "Identification of Feelings").

Session 2: Exploring Anger Feelings

> *Overview of Activities:*
>
> 1. Review of Session 1
> 2. Identifying anger feelings
> 3. Distinguish between feelings and behaviours
> 4. Benefits of managing anger
> 5. Summary

1. *WELCOME* the group.

2. *REVIEW OF SESSION 1*.

3. *IDENTIFYING ANGER FEELINGS*. Teach the group how to identify feelings of anger using the "Feelings Meter" (Figure 1) and the "Anger Signals" worksheet. The "Feelings Meter" is used to teach range of anger feelings, while the "Anger Signals" worksheet is used to teach warning signals of anger.

4. *DISTINGUISHING BETWEEN FEELINGS AND BEHAVIOURS*. Teach the group to distinguish between feelings and behaviours. Tell the group that anger is normal and appropriate, but how one expresses the feeling makes the behaviour acceptable or unacceptable.

5. *BENEFITS OF MANAGING ANGER*. Conclude the session with a discussion on the benefits of managing anger. Use the "Feelings, Behaviours and Consequences" worksheet to facilitate discussion.

6. *CONCLUSION*. Conclude meeting with a summary of what the group has learnt about the identification of feelings of anger in themselves. Encourage children to attempt the "What happens when I am angry?" worksheet as part of their homework.

Session 2
Exploring Anger Feelings

1. *Review of Session 1*

    ■   The facilitator reviews with group members what was learnt in the previous session. The children can freely recall topics discussed in Session 1 or seek clarification from the facilitator regarding specific content covered.

    ■   This will also be a good time to check group members' understanding of group rules and expectations.

2. *Explore Range of Anger Feelings*

    ■   In this segment, the facilitator teaches children how to identify feelings of anger. Drawing from concepts learnt in Session 1 on intensity of feelings, help children understand that anger feelings can range from mild (e.g., irritable), to moderate (e.g., frustrated) or severe (e.g., enraged). Use the "Feelings Meter" (see Figure 1) as a visual aid to help the child chart what makes him/her upset and what calms him/her down. The facilitator can help the child articulate the people, places or things that make him/her angry. For example, certain situations can make the child feel mildly irritated and other situations can make the child feel enraged. Likewise, there are people, places or things that can help children calm down.

    ■   Learning to recognise when one is angry involves a clear understanding of the various body, thought and action signals that serve as emotional indicators. Explain to the child that most intense feelings have three types of associated signals: a physical signal, a thought signal and an action signal.

■ The common signals for anger are as follows:

Physical Signals	Thought Signals	Action Signals
Increased pulse rate	"I hate him"	Scream/Yell/Cry
Increased rate of breathing	"I feel like breaking something"	Hit/Kick
Flushed face	"I'm going to punch her"	Threaten
Tensed muscles	"I don't ever do anything right"	Tremble
Body feels "hot" or "warm"	"I hate myself"	Withdraw

■ The facilitator can discuss with group members about times they were upset and which of these signals applied during those situations. The facilitator can use the "Anger Signals" worksheet to help group members learn about their anger signals. The facilitator might model some of these anger signals and then have the child role play what tense muscles might look like when one is angry. For older children, the facilitator can initiate a discussion about how we know what we are feeling. Appropriate initial discussion questions are "How does your body tell you when you are angry?" or "What goes through your head when you're feeling frustrated?"

3. *Distinguish Between Feelings and Behaviour*

■ The goal of this section is for group members to understand the distinction between feelings and behaviour. Specifically, the facilitator will guide the children's understanding that feelings influence but do not dictate our behaviour. This distinction is extremely important. Many children who have behavioural problems do not distinguish between their behaviour and the accompanying emotions. For example, an aggressive child will often justify his/her aggressive behaviour by explaining why he/she was angry, not recognising that feeling anger and expressing it as two separate and independent issues.

■ The facilitator will generate discussion topics which emphasise that feelings tell us how we feel like acting, but the decision of how we act is still our own. In addition, the facilitator guides the group members to understand that intense feelings such as anger are normal and appropriate, but how one expresses the feeling makes the behaviour acceptable (e.g., talking it over calmly with the offending party) or unacceptable (e.g., physically hurting the offending party).

- The facilitator can begin the discussion by having the children provide information on what they feel like doing when a certain emotion is felt (e.g., happy, sad, angry, jealous or excited). Next, the facilitators can ask what each participant generally does when he or she feels a certain emotion (e.g., anger). Without being judgmental, the facilitator will then ask the children why they do what they do when they are angry. The discussion will generally lead to children saying that they act the way they do because "they want to" or because "they just feel like it". The facilitator will then challenge the children and guide their understanding in that our emotions may make us feel a certain way, but the decision about how to act ultimately still belong to our minds (i.e., children can still think before they act). A common challenging question is, "I know you feel like cursing or throwing something, but *could* you do something else *if* you wanted to?"

- In general, during discussions, honesty from children should be encouraged because merely obtaining socially desirable/acceptable responses from these children will not assist in their development of a less negative, more prosocial orientation.

4. *Consequences of Anger*

- In this section, the facilitator can generate a discussion on the possible consequences of anger. The facilitator can use the "Feelings, Behaviours, and Consequences" worksheet to help group members see the benefits of managing their anger. Children are asked to come up with a list of advantages and disadvantages of expressing anger in an unacceptable manner.

- The facilitator will then guide the children to evaluate their decisions and to help them recognise the benefits of managing their anger.

- An example of an activity that can facilitate the children's understanding of the various consequences of anger is the "Balloon Exercise". Children will be asked to inflate a balloon, tie a knot in it, and try to explode it by squeezing it or pricking it with a sharp object. The facilitator can discuss briefly how the children felt; themes elicited can include feeling scared, angry, etc. The children will then inflate the next balloon, but this time, they will deflate the balloon by slowly releasing the air. The facilitator can then debrief the group by highlighting that the air in the balloon represents the anger they might experience. They can choose to let go of it in an explosive (i.e., negative consequence) or in an acceptable manner (i.e., positive consequence).

5. *Summary*

- The facilitator concludes the session with a summary of what the children learnt regarding anger feelings. Explain to the children that while anger is a normal feeling and that it is okay to feel angry, it is:

    a) NOT OKAY to hurt oneself when angry;

    b) NOT OKAY to hurt/hit others (including animals) when angry; and   **3 Anger Rules**

    c) NOT OKAY to destroy things when angry.

- Homework:

    Encourage children to practise identifying their anger feelings as part of their homework using the "What Happens When I Am Angry?" worksheet.

Session 3: Anger-Coping Techniques I

> *Overview of Activities:*
>
> 1. Review of Session 2
> 2. Anger-coping strategies
>   - Deep Breathing
>   - Visualisation
>   - Leisure activities
>   - Tense-and-relax (optional)
> 3. Summary

1. *WELCOME* the group.

2. *REVIEW OF SESSION 2.*

3. *INTRODUCTION TO ANGER-COPING TECHNIQUES I.* Teach the group that they can use various strategies to cope with angry situations. Tell the group that these techniques are quick, simple and effective. Link this to Session 2: Benefits of managing one's anger.

4. *DEEP BREATHING.* Introduce deep breathing to the group and explain that this technique is used by many great athletes, actors and singers around the world to calm themselves down. Role-playing techniques will also be used.

5. *VISUALISATION.* Explain visualisation to the group. Tell the group that they can calm themselves down by imagining a pleasant or peaceful scenery. Share that it would be very difficult to be angry when one is imagining him/herself engaging in an enjoyable activity.

6. *REHEARSAL OF DEEP BREATHING AND VISUALISATION.* Have the group practise using two techniques simultaneously. Play

some soothing music during this activity. Generate a discussion on their experiences using these two techniques.

7. *LEISURE ACTIVITIES*. Introduce leisure activities by telling the group that they could do other positive things to calm themselves down.

8. *TENSE-AND-RELAX (optional)*. Explain the tense-and-relax strategy to the group. Tell the group that they can calm themselves down and reduce some of the anger signals by tensing and relaxing their muscles. Link this to Session 2: Identifying Anger Feelings (anger signals). Role-playing techniques will also be used.

9. *CONCLUSION*. Conclude the session with a summary of the anger-coping techniques taught. Encourage the group to try these techniques when they encounter angry situations as part of their homework. Share with the group that they will be learning more anger-coping techniques in the next session.

Session 3
Anger-Coping Techniques I

1. *Review of Session 2*

   ■ The facilitator reviews with group members what was learnt in Session 2. The children can freely recall topics discussed in Session 2 or seek clarification from the facilitator regarding specific content covered.

2. *Anger-Coping Strategies*

   ■ Three strategies will be reviewed in this session. Facilitators have the flexibility to teach and discuss a few or all of the strategies where appropriate. Each strategy can be used on their own or in combination with other suggested strategies as aids to help the child manage his/her anger or cope with difficult situations.

   ■ **Breathing and relaxation.** Children can be taught how to breathe in and exhale slowly. Calm, deep breathing tends to have a slow rate, and stressful breathing, a more rapid one. Routines designed to lengthen the respiratory cycle will tend to have a calming effect. Slowing the breathing rate does not mean that more air is taken in or released; it means that the air travels at a slower pace. Counting strategies (e.g., count from 1 to 10 as the child exhales) lengthen the breathing cycle either by extending the breath out or by holding the breath. This technique can be made to sound important by telling children that many great athletes, rock stars and singers around the world use this simple technique to calm themselves down when they are nervous or angry. To illustrate the usefulness of this technique, the facilitator can provide an example by asking children what happens in a soccer game when a player gets very angry because of a foul committed and hits another player. Children will likely reply that the player will either be given a yellow card or a red card and get sent off the field immediately. Ask participants how different the scenario would be if the player had used deep breathing. Underscore the importance of managing our emotions and reiterate that both pleasant and unpleasant feelings are acceptable and appropriate but how we react to those feelings makes an action acceptable or unacceptable. The use of calm and deep breathing can be a useful tool in helping the child manage his/her intense emotions. The facilitator can use the "Deep Breathing" script (see Appendix 4) to help group members remember this technique.

- **Visualisation and relaxation.** Relaxation usually goes hand in hand with visualisation because relaxation is generally considered a precondition as well as an effect of visualisation. The child can be instructed to build an imaginary scene or a special place as a retreat for relaxation. The scene should be rich in sensory images of sight, sound, taste, smell, texture and even temperature. The child is instructed to imagine that the body feels progressively more relaxed. Some children prefer to visualise a special indoor place such as an attic room, while others prefer to visualise outdoor places such as the beach. Use the "Visualisation" script (see Appendix 4) to help the child imagine a peaceful and pleasant place. Another suggestion is for the child to imagine a huge balloon filled with helium weighed down by heavy bags of concrete. Each bag of concrete represents a different problem that the child is struggling with. Have the child visualise that these bags of concrete drop off one at a time until the balloon is able to float feely in the sky.

- **Leisure Activities.** Children can be taught to engage in some positive alternative action to cope effectively with anger or frustration. Some alternatives that children can do include being involved in sports (e.g., jogging, swimming and playing basketball), music (e.g., playing an instrument, singing and listening to music), or creative arts (e.g., drawing, painting, writing and dancing). The facilitator can choose to introduce this segment by asking the children to list some fun activities that they can do to calm themselves down when they are feeling upset. After the children have done that, facilitators can integrate all children's responses and compile a list of positive activities generated by the group. For younger children, instead of having them write, they could draw some positive things they do to help themselves become less agitated or angry.

- **Tense-and-Relax (optional).** The tense-and-relax method or commonly known as progressive muscle relaxation (PMR) is a common component in the treatment of behavioural problems among children (e.g., Kellner, Bry, & Salvador, 2008; Sukhodolsky et al., 2009; Weisz & Gray, 2008). The use of PMR has been associated with various physiological and psychological benefits such as lowered blood pressure, heart rate, anxiety and physical tension (Conrad Krajewski, Sauerland, & Wieland, 2011; Dolbier & Taylor, 2012). Getting the muscles to tense and then relax can help reduce some of physiological signals associated with anger. Explain to the children that the tense-and-relax strategy allows their bodies to release tension and anger by tightening certain muscle groups at a time. Use the "Tense-and-Relax" script (see Appendix 4) to help children practise tensing and relaxing their muscles.

3. *Summary*

- The facilitator concludes the session with a summary of what the children learned regarding the above-mentioned anger-coping strategies.

- *Homework:*

    a) Encourage children to practice one or more of the anger-coping strategies (see "My Practice Diary" worksheet for Session 3).

    b) As part of their homework, encourage children to attempt to use one or more of the positive coping strategies learnt when they encounter problematic situations or when someone makes them angry (See "My Coping Diary" worksheet for Session 3).

Session 4: Anger-Coping Techniques II

> *Overview of Activities:*
>
> 1. Review of Session 3 and homework
> 2. Anger-coping strategies
>   - Being firm
>   - Social support
>   - Happy thoughts
>   - Story-telling (optional)
> 3. Summary

1. *WELCOME* the group.

2. *REVIEW OF SESSION 3 AND HOMEWORK.*

3. *INTRODUCTION TO ANGER-COPING TECHNIQUES II.* Teach the group a few or all of the strategies where appropriate using the **FISH** acronym — being **FI**rm, **S**ocial support and **H**appy thoughts.

4. *BEING FIRM.* Tell the group that an assertive person states his/her stand without being obnoxious, aggressive or too passive, by being polite and maintaining eye contact with the person he/she is talking to.

5. *HAPPY THOUGHTS.* Introduce the group to happy thoughts by telling them that they could say these statements to calm themselves down in an emotionally intense situation.

6. *SOCIAL SUPPORT.* Explain to the group that it might be a good idea to ask someone for help when encountering a problematic situation that they cannot solve on their own.

7. *STORY-TELLING (optional).* Introduce story-telling techniques to the group. Each group member and facilitator will take

turns to tell a story. Alternatively, both the group and facilitator can take turns to write down their story.

8. *CONCLUSION*. Conclude the session with a summary of the anger-coping techniques taught. Encourage the group to try these techniques when they encounter angry situations as part of their homework. Share with the group that they will be learning perspective-taking skills next week.

Session 4
Anger-Coping Techniques II

1. *Review of Session 3 and Homework*

   ■ The facilitator reviews what was learnt in Session 3 by discussing the homework assignment. In particular, it is helpful to review which of the strategies and techniques the children found helpful and which of these did not work for them. Facilitators should also explore with the children possible reasons why certain techniques and strategies did not work well for them.

2. *Anger-Coping Strategies*

   ■ Four strategies will be reviewed in this session. Facilitators have the flexibility to teach and discuss a few or all of the strategies where appropriate. Each strategy can be used on their own or in combination with other suggested strategies as aids to help the child manage his/her anger or cope with difficult situations. The FISH acronym (being **FI**rm, **S**ocial support and **H**appy thoughts) can be used to help children remember the anger-coping strategies taught in this session.

   ■ **Being Firm.** Children can be taught to make requests and refusals calmly and assertively, not passively or aggressively. An assertive person states his/her stand without being obnoxious, aggressive or too passive. Children can be taught the following:

     — Standing up for oneself does not mean getting back at someone else.

     — Standing up for oneself does not mean acting obnoxiously or in a bossy manner.

     — Standing up for oneself does not mean saying or doing anything at anytime.

- The "FIRM" worksheet can be used to help group members learn some of the assertiveness techniques stated below:

  — The use of "I" statements

  — Stating feelings and needs

  — Giving and receiving compliments

  — Refusing

  — Making and accepting negative requests

  — Be polite and respectful

  — Maintain eye contact

- Communication is a complex endeavour. Because of aggressive children's social-cognitive deficits, they do not perceive and interpret messages accurately, and often resort to using manipulative and/or violent means to get what they want. Teaching these children the need to use "I" statements more frequently to express their feelings and needs would facilitate clear and functional communication which would in turn minimise the chances of conversational exchanges going awry. Singaporeans, like other Asians, appear to be awkward when receiving compliments. For example when a compliment is given the recipient would typically respond with a denial (e.g., "No, actually, it's not that good."). Children can learn to accept a compliment gracefully, and say "thank you" when a compliment is given. In addition, children can also learn that positive expressions can foster good social skills. They do not need for others to do something for them before they say something complimentary. For example, when a child notices that her classmate seated next to her has done drawn a beautiful picture during Art class, she can learn to say, "Hey Siti, that's really good!" Children also need to be taught refusal skills. Sometimes, to be accepted by peers, children will violate rules or manifest a variety of problem behaviours ranging from showing off to truancy or using illicit drugs. Teaching refusal skills is best accomplished by planning, rehearsing and role-playing these skills. The child can learn to say "No thanks, I don't smoke" and walk away when peers offer him/her a cigarette. When teaching refusal skills, facilitators may want to also discuss with children the potential consequences of submitting to peer pressure. With a younger child, this involves discussing how certain behaviours will get him/her into trouble. With older children, the facilitators might want to take the discussion further, and discuss how certain actions might make someone else feel. Children will also need to learn that they may not always be successful in having their requests granted, but making requests (whether positive or negative) in an assertive manner will pay off more frequently than passive or aggressive behaviour. They will need to learn that in the course of interacting with others, it is inevitable that they will occasionally offend others, and it is better idea to accept the fact that they are in the wrong rather than to counter-attack. Being polite and respectful are important aspects of effective communication. Children could demonstrate politeness and respect to the person whom they are talking to by expressing themselves in a tone that is calm and not threatening. In addition, children need to learn to maintain eye contact with the person whom they are interacting with. Eye contact indicates one's attention and respect for both listener and speaker.

- **Social Support.** Sometimes children may encounter a problematic or angry situation that they cannot solve on their own. In such situations, asking someone for help is a wise thing to do. Because aggressive children are often rejected by their peers, it may be difficult for them to know who they can approach for help. Therefore, helping them identify a social support network would be helpful (e.g., parent, teacher, sibling, a friend, etc.). In addition, it would also be helpful to teach them the right time to ask for help by evaluating the seriousness of the situation. For instance, if the situation is not so serious, teach the child that he/she can choose to deal with the situation him/herself by using the anger-coping techniques or ask the person for help when he/she is available. If the situation is quite serious, ask the person for help when he/she is free. If the situation is very serious, ask the person for help immediately. Another important aspect is to teach the child to express clearly as to how he/she wants the person to help. For example, teach the child that he/she could ask the person to help him/her feel better by talking to him/her or giving a hug or to help him/her solve the problem. The "Social Support" worksheet can be used to help children learn this strategy.

- **Happy Thoughts.** These are positive coping statements that children can say to themselves (thoughts) to calm themselves down and help themselves cope with their anger or with an emotionally intense situation. The "Happy Thoughts" worksheet can be used to help group members learn some positive coping statements. Some examples include the following:

  — "Stay relaxed ... take it easy."

  — "Stay cool... I'm going be OK."

  — "It's not worth fighting over this. That guy's going be the one ending up looking silly, I'm the smart one."
  — "Forget it! That's wasting my energy and time... my heart is pumping harder than it needs to be."
  — "That's OK... I'll just let him continue to shout and scream, and if I don't retaliate and if I don't react angrily, he'll end up looking like a fool!"

Aggressive children often view not fighting back as being weak, passive or cowardly. Facilitators should challenge the participants' view of physical or mental strength. Explain to the participants that reacting calmly to an angry person or situation is actually a more difficult response than to react explosively in return. The analogy of the automatic knee-jerk response can be used. When the knee is tapped below the patella, the knee-jerk reflex occurs, and this response does not require any conscious planning or thought. Conversely, if one were to attempt to stop the knee jerk-reflex, it would prove rather difficult. Reacting in a verbally or physically aggressive manner comes almost automatically to aggressive children and that can be analogous to the knee jerk response which is relatively easy and essentially does not require thought. On the other hand, if the child were to react calmly in a difficult situation, he/she would have demonstrated self-control which is a far more difficult response.

- **Story-telling.** Story-telling techniques have been recommended for use with aggressive, oppositional and acting-out children (e.g., Harris & Walton, 2009; Nicolopoulou, 2007; Smith, 2009). Stories are a way of communicating with children on a metaphorical level. Because stories deal with other people, this technique provides some degree of emotional distancing which allows children to minimise their defences and become more receptive to the indirect message conveyed. This activity is played with the child and facilitator taking turns to tell stories. Children randomly select a card from a stack of cards (see Appendix 5) which contains an emotionally arousing word or phrase such as "punch", "argue" or "failed the final exam". The child will have to tell a story that contains the word or phrase that appears on the card selected. After the child has finished telling the story, it is the facilitator's turn to tell his/her story based on the same word or phrase. The facilitator's story must contain elements similar to the story told by the child, but he/she needs to draw a lesson or moral from the story as experienced by the protagonist. Facilitators should not directly instruct the child about the lesson to be learnt or it would defeat the usefulness of this technique. Instead, the facilitator should state the moral or lesson learnt through the eyes of the protagonist. This way, the facilitator is indirectly teaching and directing the child to find the solutions to the protagonist's problems which the child could also use in his/her life. Alternatively, instead of the facilitator re-telling the story, both the child and facilitator can take turns to write down their story.

3. *Summary*

    ■   The facilitator concludes the session with a summary of what the children learnt on the above-mentioned anger-coping strategies.

    ■   Homework:

        Encourage children to practise one or more of the anger coping strategies (see "My Practice Diary" worksheet for Session 4).

Session 5: Empathy Skills

> *Overview of Activities:*
>
> 1. Review of Session 4 and homework
> 2. Building empathy
> 3. Summary

1. *WELCOME* the group.

2. *REVIEW OF SESSION 4 AND HOMEWORK.*

3. *BUILDING EMPATHY.* Teach the group that empathy is the ability to understand and recognise others' feelings, and that they can hurt others through their behaviour.

4. *CONCLUSION.* Encourage the group to practice empathy skills in a problematic situation as these skills would help them think ahead before acting out certain behaviours. Also, tell the group that they will be learning perspective-taking skills next week.

Session 5
Empathy Skills

1. *Review of Session 4 and Homework*

   ▪ The facilitator reviews what was learnt in Session 4 by discussing the homework assignment. In particular, it is helpful to review which of the strategies and techniques the participants found helpful and which of these did not work for them. Facilitators should also explore with the participants the possible reasons why certain techniques and strategies did not work well for them.

2. *Building Empathy*

   ▪ This section deals with building empathy skills in children. Empathy can be defined as the understanding of another's emotional state, the sharing of another's emotional state and the prosocial behaviours that follow (Dadds et al., 2008; Eisenberg, Spinrad, & Sadovsky, 2006; Hoffman, 2000).

   ▪ The facilitator can start with teaching the children empathy by using the "Everyone Has Feelings" worksheet to help group members develop the ability to decode and label emotions of another. Facilitators should select appropriate scenarios to discuss with group members or to use all scenarios depending on the age of the child or children, and composition of children involved. Facilitators are advised to use their discretion in the choice of scenarios in order to maximise the productivity of the discussion. Following that, the facilitator can move on to guiding the children through the "Practising Empathy" worksheet.

   ▪ An important point to highlight during this session is the importance of having empathy. Children often do not understand why they have to step into the affective world of other people. A simple discussion may help internalise the need to be empathetic. The facilitator can get the group to generate and brainstorm the reasons to have empathy (e.g., so they would not hurt their loved ones, so they have the ability to understand their friends' actions better or help them better).

■ Another important focus of this session is to highlight to the children that sometimes they may only think of their own feelings and forget that other people have feelings as well. Explain to the children how they can sometimes unknowingly hurt others through their behaviours. The "Consequences of Showing Empathy" worksheet can be used to generate discussion during this segment. During the discussion, get the children to ask themselves the following questions:

o What is the problem? Or what is my behaviour like?

o How does the person feel? Why?

o What can I do to make the person feel better?

■ If necessary, the facilitator can end off the session by distinguishing between empathy and sympathy. Children often confuse the idea of empathy with sympathy. Sympathy can be defined as feeling sorry for someone and wanting the person to feeling happier and/or better. This is a different concept to how empathy is construed.

■ The facilitator may consider using the "Darer" and "Performer" activity to help children further understand the need to be empathetic. First, pair the children in groups of two. Assign one child to be the "Darer" and the other to be the "Performer". Brief the "Darers" in a separate room and explain that they need to come up with a task for their partner (the "Performer") to carry out. The facilitator at this juncture may set certain limits to the task (e.g., no vulgarities). However, the facilitator should not give any reminders to the child with regard to being empathetic. Following that, the "Darers" will announce their tasks in front of the group and the "Performers" will be asked to carry out the given task. The facilitator will supervise the execution of the task. After completion of the tasks, the facilitator will invite the "Darers" and the "Performers" to share how they felt (e.g., whether the "Performers" felt reluctant to carry out the tasks, whether the "Darers" thought twice about asking their partners to perform certain tasks, etc.). The main focus of this discussion is to elicit responses and/or foster the children to have empathy towards their peers by thinking ahead how they might feel if they were made to do an embarrassing task. The facilitator should find the opportunity to bridge how sometimes one might have a lot of fun but neglect to be mindful of what the other person might feel.

3. *Summary*

- The facilitator concludes the session with a summary of what the children learnt on empathy skills.

- Homework:

  Encourage children to practise empathy skills (see "Consequences of Showing Empathy" worksheet). The facilitator should generate other situations that are relevant to the children.

Session 6: Perspective-Taking Skills

Overview of Activities:

1. Review of Session 5 and homework
2. Perspective-taking
3. Summary

1. *WELCOME* the group.

2. *REVIEW OF SESSION 5 AND HOMEWORK.*

3. *PERSPECTIVE-TAKING.* Teach the group that perspective-taking is a skill that enables us to understand a situation from another person's view. Guide the group members to understand that not all negative social encounters are necessarily motivated by hostile intent. Help them learn how not to misinterpret their peers' intent and jump to a false conclusion before evaluating all the relevant facts.

4. *CONCLUSION.* Encourage the group to practise perspective-taking skills in a problematic situation as these skills would help them think ahead before acting out certain behaviours. Also, tell the group that they will be learning "Fighting Fair" next week.

Session 6
Perspective-Taking Skills

1. *Review of Session 5 and Homework*

   ▪ The facilitator reviews what was learnt in Session 5 by discussing the homework assignment. Children need to recognise that they can hurt others through their actions.

2. *Situation Interpretation and Perspective-Taking in Ambiguous Situations*

   ▪ **Perspective-Taking.** The goal of this session is to help the children understand that there are many ways of seeing and interpreting the same thing. The facilitator can guide the children to see things from both their point of view as well as those of others. Seeing another person's point of view is also known as perspective-taking. Perspective-taking is important because it allows the children to understand a situation from another person's point of view. The facilitator can choose to use an activity that uses visual illusion pictures to help children understand the concept of perspective-taking. Have each child look at the selected visual illusion picture and write on a piece of paper what he/she sees without looking at what others have written. Once they have written a response, ask each child to state what he/she perceived the picture to be. Generate a group discussion on why everyone looked at the same picture but yet each person could have seen different things. This activity can be repeated with other visual illusion pictures if needed.

   ▪ Explain to the children that perspective-taking is important in helping them to manage their angry feelings in negative social situations. It can help them understand that sometimes, a person's negative behaviour is not motivated by bad intentions. It is important for the facilitator to emphasise the need to learn how to interpret another person's intention and not jump to a false conclusion before checking out all the relevant facts. It is almost like being a good detective looking for evidence before catching the right culprit.

- Materials and resources for this section can be found in Appendices 6 and 7. There are a total of six vignettes. The descriptions of the vignettes and instructions for the facilitator can be found in Appendix 6. Appendix 7 contains pictures that accompany selected vignettes. Each vignette has three accompanying pictures. Facilitators have the option of discussing a couple or all of the vignettes. While discussing these vignettes, the facilitator can ask the group to write their responses in the "Perspective-Taking" worksheet. The description of these vignettes and pictures were first developed by Hughes (1996). Because of cultural differences, these vignettes and pictures have been adapted for use in the Singapore context.

- Aggressive children having a tendency to misinterpret others' benign behaviour as being hostile in intent, and would typically construe any ambiguous situation in a negative light. For example, looking at the discussion questions and pictures provided in Appendices 6 and 7, aggressive children's responses will usually reflect a belief that the child either deliberately hit him/her with the ball or purposefully knocked into him/her causing his/her lunch to spill all over the floor.

- The purpose of this section is for the facilitator to guide the discussion in such a way that the child gradually recognises the possibility that these negative social encounters (e.g., hit by the ball or splashed with mud) could be the result of an accident. A high level of skill is required of the facilitator to steer the discussion in the needed direction.

- An example is provided using Vignette 1. In the following exchange, 'C' represents 'child' and 'F' represents 'facilitator'.

F: What do you think happened? Why do you think he hit you with the ball?

C: I don't know… I think he did it purposely. He took this chance to hit me with the ball when my back was facing him.

F: Really? How far away do you think this other boy was from where you were?

C: I don't know... but look … he's not even throwing the ball in a straight line. He's aiming the ball at me.

F: Yeah, I *suppose* there *might be a possibility* that he *could have* hit you deliberately. Let's pretend that the two boys were playing quite close to the monkey bars where you were. *Is it possible* that the ball hit you by accident because the two boys were playing so close to the monkey bars?

C: No … I tell you, he purposely did it! He's not blind!

F: OK, I'm going to give you two different scenarios. I want you to tell me in which scenario would it be *more likely* that the boy deliberately hit you with the ball. The first scenario is when the two boys are playing very far away from the monkey bars, maybe some 50 metres away, and the ball hits you. The second scenario is when the two boys are playing nearby, maybe less than 5 metres away and the ball hits you. If both scenarios happened to you, in which of the scenarios do you think it *might have been accidental* and in which of the scenarios do you think it *might have been deliberate*?

C: I think if the two boys are playing nearby and I got hit, it could be accidental. But if I got hit when they are playing very far away, then I think it's probably done on purpose.

F: Let's pretend again, OK? Let's pretend that this time, the boy who threw the ball that hit you actually wears very thick spectacles. He has short-sightedness of maybe 900 degrees in his right eye and 800 degrees in his left eye. Unfortunately, today, he forgot to bring his spectacles but still felt like playing in the field even though he couldn't see very well. In this situation, *could it be possible* that it was not done on purpose? That it was an accident?

C: Yeah, I guess so.

- Leading the discussion in a manner that the child gradually comes to recognise that not all negative social encounters are necessarily motivated by hostile intent will not be an easy task. There are a few important points to take note. The facilitator will need to creatively and spontaneously generate alternative situations with facts incompatible with hostile intent, thus teaching children to pay attention to cues that are inconsistent with hostile intent. These activities will help children learn how not to misinterpret their peers' intent and jump to a false conclusion before assessing all the relevant facts. It is also important for facilitators not to disagree with children who insist that these negative acts are purposefully done. Rather, in responding to the child, the facilitator can restate the child's answer in tentative terms as exemplified by the italicised portions of the verbal exchange between the facilitator and the child based on Vignette 1. This is because some acts could indeed be performed with malicious intent and it is <u>not</u> the purpose of this programme to teach children that all actions always either have positive or benign intent. The objective is to teach children to carefully examine all cues (not merely focusing exclusively on hostile ones) so as not to leap to a wrong conclusion.

- Most aggressive children will generate responses that reflect an exclusive focus on hostile cues, thus attributing malicious intent to others in ambiguous situations. However, on occasion, you will encounter some children who appear to understand, in varying degrees, the importance of analysing all available cues in the environment prior to coming to a conclusion. If this were the case, the facilitator's role becomes less complex. The facilitator can then discuss with the child the types of circumstances, situations and cues that might be perceived to contain or not contain hostile intent.

■ It is also important to generate discussion on how the children might feel if they perceive an act to be performed with malicious intent (i.e., on purpose) or benign intent (i.e., accidental). Typically, one might feel more angry or upset if he/she perceives the act to be done on purpose than when it is accidental. Lead the discussion in a manner that children gradually understand that they can better manage their angry feelings when they analyse all available cues in the environment prior to coming to a conclusion.

■ As a final point, the facilitator can emphasise the difference between perspective-taking and empathy (learnt in Session 5). Highlight that empathy refers to putting themselves into another person's shoes and trying to understand how he/she might be *feeling*. On the other hand, perspective-taking refers to trying to understand a situation from another person's point of view and figure out what he/she might be *thinking*.

3. *Summary*

■ The facilitator concludes the session with a summary of what the children learnt on perspective-taking skills.

■ Homework:

Encourage children to practise perspective-taking skills (see worksheet on "Perspective-Taking"). The facilitator can opt to use the suggested vignettes (see above) or to generate other vignettes that are relevant to the children.

Session 7: Fighting Fair

Overview of Activities:

1. Review of Session 6 and homework
2. Fighting Fair
3. Activities for Fighting Fair
4. Summary

1. *WELCOME* the group.

2. *REVIEW OF SESSION 6 AND HOMEWORK*.

3. *FIGHTING FAIR*. Teach the group that "Fighting Fair" is a process of working out differences or disagreements during an argument in which individuals attack the problem and not the person. Using "Fighting Fair" would enable them to resolve frustration and conflict in a healthy manner without hurting the relationship or those involved.

4. *ACTIVITIES FOR FIGHTING FAIR*. Get the group to practise "Fighting Fair" using the role play cards provided in Appendix 8. Discuss and process the role-playing with the group.

5. *CONCLUSION*. Encourage the group to practice the "Fighting Fair" technique in a problematic situation as part of their homework. Tell the group that they will be learning Prosocial Skills next week.

Session 7
Fighting Fair

1. *Review of Session 6 and Homework*

   ■ The facilitator reviews what was learnt in Session 6, focusing on the fact that negative social encounters may or may not contain malicious intent. It is critical that participants learn how to discern cues that are associated with hostile and non-hostile intent.

2. *Fighting Fair*

   ■ "Fighting Fair" was first used by McKay, Rogers and McKay (1989) for teaching couples to deal with conflict, but this technique can be adapted for use with children.

   ■ The facilitator can choose to begin this session with the "Who Has the Tallest Tower?" activity. Divide the children into two groups and tell them that they are required to build a tower of cards with a set of materials chosen within a pre-set time limit (e.g., 5 min). The group with the tallest tower wins. The groups should be unevenly divided (e.g., a group of three versus a group of two). There should also be a markedly unfair distribution of materials (e.g., one group with a roll of scotchtape and the other group with a small piece of tape). After the activity has concluded, generate discussion on how the children think and feel about the game. Ask questions like:

     — How did the game make you feel?

     — What does 'fair' mean to you?

     — How can you make the game fairer?

   ■ To stimulate responses, direct the discussion for the children to understand that it is important to play fair and resolve any conflict in an amicable manner. Without which, they might be left feeling upset or unjust. The facilitator should consider the responses from the children and lead the discussion appropriately.

■ Next, the facilitator can share with the children that conflict exists in all relationships, and experiencing conflict does not necessarily lead to aggression or loss of control. Explain to the children that sometimes people have disagreements in their ideas or what they want to do. An example of a disagreement is when he/she and his/her friend want to play different games. For instance, he may want to play Monopoly, while his friend may want to play computer games. Such a disagreement may lead both individuals feeling angry or upset and may even end up in a fight. So, how can both of them resolve this disagreement without getting into a fight? This is when "Fighting Fair" comes to the rescue.

■ What is 'Fighting Fair'? It is the process of working out differences or disagreements during an argument in which individuals attack the problem and not the person. The underlying concept of "Fighting Fair" assumes that we do not communicate clearly when we are angry. "Fighting Fair" is a method of resolving frustration and conflict by building rather than tearing down relationships, and it allows anger to be expressed in a healthy way. "Fighting Fair" can be used at home, in school or any time that children are involved in a fight.

■ Use the "What Is Fighting Fair?" worksheet to teach the five rules for Fighting Fair. The facilitator can use the Mr CRAWL acronym to help the children remember the five rules:

a) **C**are for the other person's feelings

b) Be **R**esponsible for your own actions

c) **A**void "fouls"

d) **W**hat is the problem? Attack the problem, not the person

e) **L**isten to the other person, and allow for disagreement

- **Care for the other person's feelings.** It is important that children learn to be sensitive to the feelings of others. One way to do this is to use caring language as part of their communication even when they are angry. Caring language is language that is non-threatening and communicates respect. Also, use a non-threatening tone of voice when speaking.

- **Be responsible for your own actions.** When children are in an argument or in a fight, they often do not see how they contribute to the problem. They tend to blame others. Blaming other people is an example of not taking responsibility for one's actions. Each person involved in the argument or fight should ask, "How did I contribute to this problematic situation, and what can I do to handle this problem?"

- **Avoid "fouls".** A "foul" is any tool which causes conflict to escalate. Some "fouls" include hitting, pushing, blaming, threatening, name-calling, taking revenge, not listening and excuse-giving. Examples of statements involving "fouls" include "It's all your fault", "You are so stupid. you never do anything right", and "Don't blame me, Xiaoming did it".

- **What is the problem?** Attack the problem, not the person. Very frequently, when children encounter conflict situations, they have a tendency not to focus on the problem and begin blaming the other person. Children can be taught to remain focused on the issue at hand even though their emotions are running high.

- **Listen to the other person, and allow for disagreement.** Facilitators can teach children not to interrupt the other person and to ask questions if he/she is unclear. Children can also be reminded not to complete other people's sentences for them; allow other people to speak for themselves. Children must learn to allow for disagreement — disagreeing with someone does not mean that a fight need necessarily ensue.

3. *Fighting Fair Learning Activities*

- At this point, participants would have learnt how to fight fair using the five "Fighting Fair" rules. Facilitators can proceed with giving the children an opportunity to practise "Fighting Fair" using the role-playing cards provided in the appendices. Appendix 8 provides role-playing cards for children. Facilitators may choose to utilise all or a sample of the role-playing cards as deemed appropriate.

- Participants will be asked to find someone in the group to role-play with them. Alternatively, the teacher or counsellor can pair the participants up. Facilitators can choose to select a couple of role-play scenarios for the children or have different pairs of children role play different scenarios. The final decision regarding how best to conduct these "Fighting Fair" activities lies with the facilitator. The important issue is that children are given an opportunity to put into practice what they have learnt about "Fighting Fair" through the materials provided.

- Finally, after the role-playing, the teacher or counsellor should discuss and process the role-plays with the class or group as a whole. Was it difficult for the children to do the role plays within the "constraints" of "Fighting Fair" rules? Which rule did they feel was hardest to follow? Allow children and adolescents to share how they felt as they did their role-plays. It is crucial for participants to learn how to solve problems without hurting another person's feelings and without resorting to verbal or physical aggression. Besides learning through teacher- or counsellor-led discussions, participants can also appreciate appropriate problem-solving approaches from each other. Even when facilitators are working with individual children, it remains important for facilitators to process the role-plays with the child.

4. *Summary*

- The facilitator concludes the session with a summary of what the children learnt on "Fighting Fair".

■   Homework:

Children are encouraged to use the "Fighting Fair" technique they have learnt in Session 7 to solve problems and resolve conflict they encounter this week as part of their homework (see "Applying Fighting Fair" worksheet).

Session 8: Building Prosocial Skills

> *Overview of Activities:*
>
> 1. Review of Session 7 and homework
> 2. Prosocial skills
> 3. Activities for building prosocial skills
> 4. Random acts of kindness
> 5. Summary

1. *WELCOME* the group.

2. *REVIEW OF SESSION 7 AND HOMEWORK.*

3. *PROSOCIAL SKILLS.* Introduce the group to prosocial skills by asking them to do the "Prosocial Skills" worksheet. Generate discussion based on the responses given by the group. Tell the group that learning these prosocial skills would enable to them to cope with social situations in a more positive manner.

4. *ACTIVITIES FOR BUILDING PROSOCIAL SKILLS.* Have the group practice prosocial skills using the Activity Cards provided in Appendix 9.

5. *RANDOM ACTS OF KINDNESS.* Introduce "Acts of Kindness" to the group. Explain to the group that an act of kindness does not have to be a huge and complex endeavour. Tell them that this act of kindness can be as simple as opening the door for someone, saying something encouraging to someone who is sad or saying thank you to someone.

6. *CONCLUSION.* Conclude the meeting with a summary of what the group has learnt on Prosocial Skills. Encourage children to attempt the "Random Act of Kindness" worksheet as part of their homework.

Session 8
Building Prosocial Skills

1. *Review of Session 7 and Homework*

   ■ Facilitators will generate a discussion cum sharing session with participants on the types of problems they encountered in which they used the "Fighting Fair" technique. Ask participants to share their experiences on how successful or unsuccessful they were when using "Fighting Fair" rules in negotiating a problematic or tricky situation. Facilitators can also share with the group or child some occasions in which they have used "Fighting Fair" rules to resolve disagreements in a friendly and peaceful manner.

2. *Building Prosocial Skills*

   ■ The facilitator introduces this session by teaching the group about the different types of prosocial skills: sharing, cooperating, helping, making friends and keeping out of fights. The "Prosocial Skills" worksheet can be used as a guide.

   ■ Following that, the facilitator can have group members participate in one or more of the following suggested activities:

   a) **Learning Prosocial Skills through Discussion Questions.** This activity is structured in a game-like format whereby each participant draws a card and responds to what is stated on the card. The Activity Cards provided in Appendix 9 can be used for this activity. Facilitators have the flexibility to choose a sample of activity cards if they feel that certain cards appear more appropriate for their group members. Activity cards can be detached by cutting along the dotted lines. Blank cards are provided for facilitators to write their own activity questions.

<u>Variation 1:</u> If this activity is to be played with a group of six to eight children, the facilitator can divide the group members into two teams. The facilitator will judge the participants' responses for appropriateness. Appropriate responses will be awarded with two tokens (e.g., one-cent coins or poker chips can be used as tokens). Responses that are judged to be less appropriate will be awarded one token. The team with the most number of tokens "wins". It is critical that the facilitator understands that the goal of this exercise is not in playing the game and winning per se. Generally, the facilitator would want to make everyone a winner. The game-like format only serves to arouse and maintain the interest of the children. The objective of this exercise is to help children become more socially aware of the world around them and to teach them some essential social skills to help them cope in a more positive manner. In the light of this, this activity need not be played following traditional game rules. For example, there can be flexibility regarding how or when to award tokens, or even how to win the game. The facilitator's aim is to shape and guide the participant's response in such a manner that the participant can earn the maximum number of tokens. The facilitator can choose to have all team members discuss and contribute towards fulfilling the activity on the activity card. If this is done, the facilitator can award a token to each contributing team member. To avoid creating a competitive atmosphere when played with two or more opposing teams, the facilitator can issue a general challenge for all participants. For example, a target goal could be set for all participants in two teams to earn a combined total of an arbitrary number of points (e.g., 18 points). This way, teams need not compete to outdo each other; rather, they can work together to achieve a common goal. It is essential that the activity be used as a platform for discussion, sharing and teaching.

Variation 2: If this activity is to be played with a class of 40 pupils, the teacher will need to divide the class into four or five groups. Each group can elect their representative to come up and draw a game card from the teacher. Each representative can then brainstorm with group members and come up with a group response. Subsequently, the teacher can judge the group response for appropriateness and award tokens accordingly.

Variation 3: This activity can be conducted as discussion questions with individual children.

b) **Learning Prosocial Skills through a Group Project.** Get the children to decide on the project they want to work on (e.g., build a monster/alien/dinosaur from recycled materials). After they have decided as a team (with minimal assistance from the facilitator) which project they want to work on and its name, tell the children that they need to pay attention to the prosocial acts others did while working on the project. For example, "I noticed John helped Tom with sticking the cardboard together" or "John came over to help me with the cutting". Give a time limit for the activity and let them begin. During the activity, the facilitator should only offer minimal intervention but pay attention to how the children resolve conflicts (if any), how they problem-solve, prosocial acts performed, etc. These will be used as discussion points later. When the activity has concluded, ask the group for prosocial acts they have observed that others did (for themselves or for other members of the group). The facilitator can also offer feedback on the prosocial acts he/she observed. Thereafter, the facilitator can bring up any problematic situation for discussion and ask the children how they can act differently, in a more prosocial manner.

3. *Random Acts of Kindness*

■ The idea 'random acts of kindness' is taken from the book *Random Acts of Kindness* (Conari Press, 2000, 2013). This book is a collection of stories about the little things that people do for one another, which inspired thousands of people to become involved in promoting kindness in their own communities.

- Many children who display behavioural difficulties have developed such a repertoire of unacceptable behaviours over many years such that these negative behaviours become almost part of these children's personality and self-image. This homework exercise is part of a powerful intervention technique to gradually reverse this negative downward spiral by deliberately putting children in situations where they will behave well and even in altruistic ways.

- It is important for the facilitator to explain to the children that an act of kindness does not have to be a huge and complex endeavour. Sometimes, children shy away from doing good because they feel that it is an unattainable goal. So it is important for facilitators to convey to children that acts of kindness required in this homework exercise are simple things people do for each other such as opening the door for someone, saying something encouraging to someone who is sad or saying thank you to someone. It is hoped that kindness will be infectious but even if it is not, each act of kindness is its own reward. Likewise, through this exercise, children will be taught to notice little deeds of kindness that others do for them on a daily basis. Many little deeds of kindness go unnoticed and this exercise hopes to raise children's awareness that acts of kindness can come in different shapes and sizes.

- The basic principle of this intervention is as follows. When children perform these acts of kindness, two things happen: a) they begin to see themselves in a more positive light, no matter how much they would rather see themselves as "bad", and b) they will be perceived by others as doing something good, and it is hoped that they would get some degree of social approval.

- Resistance from the children is to be expected. It is unlikely that angry or difficult children will readily embrace the idea of helping others or noticing the good that others do.

Generally, the more severe the behavioural problem that a child has, the more the facilitator should make a concerted effort to get the child to do and notice these acts of kindness. When doing this activity for the first couple of times, it is not necessary for the facilitator to ensure that the children have a positive attitude. Having a positive attitude towards helping others will take time to develop and will come much later. At this stage, it is more important that the "good act" gets done. The facilitator should present the homework as a "forced-choice" activity: children should not be asked *if* they want to do something, but they do have a choice as to *what* they want to do.

- Optional: Before the facilitator concludes the session, the children can be asked to think of an act of kindness they can perform right away supervised by the facilitator. For example, if the children are in a school, they can consider going to the canteen and help the canteen vendors clear any utensils that are left on the tables. This can be done as a group or individually. The children will be required to come up with their own act of kindness to perform. The facilitator can do a quick debrief on how they felt after the act of kindness was accomplished. This gives the children a chance to experience the positive reward(s) of engaging in a prosocial behaviour.

4. *Summary*

- The facilitator concludes the session with a summary of what the children learnt on Prosocial Skills.

- Homework:

  The facilitator will ask the children to do two things as part of their homework assignment (see worksheet on "Random Acts of Kindness").

a) Each child is to notice an act of kindness someone did for him/her at home, in school or in any other setting.

b) Each child is to do something positive and kind for someone they know (e.g., parent, siblings, teacher, peer or neighbour).

Session 9: Effective Problem-Solving Steps: ANGER Plan

> *Overview of Activities:*
>
> 1. Review of Session 8 and homework
> 2. ANGER plan
> 3. Summary

1. *WELCOME* the group.

2. *REVIEW OF SESSION 8 AND HOMEWORK.*

3. *INTRODUCTION TO PROBLEM-SOLVING.* Begin by asking the group for examples of situations that are problematic to them. Ask them for steps that they would normally take when they encounter such situations. Guide them to generate steps in solving such situations.

4. *ANGER PLAN.* Introduce and teach the five steps in the ANGER Plan.

5. *HOMEWORK.* Encourage the group to learn the five steps of the ANGER Plan as part of their homework.

6. *CONCLUSION.* Conclude the session by telling the group that the ANGER Plan would help them resolve their problems systematically. Finally, tell the group that they will be learning about the application of the ANGER Plan next week.

Session 9
Effective Problem-Solving Steps: ANGER Plan

1. *Review of Session 8*

   - A critical component of this review section is to process and discuss the homework assignment. The process of review and discussion of these random acts of kindness is as important as the homework itself.

   - The facilitator can generate a discussion with participants about how they feel when someone did something nice for them unexpectedly. It is also critical to explore how the children feel and react when they performed an act of kindness for someone else. Very often, it would also be helpful to ask children about the impact an act of kindness has on the recipient.

   - Sometimes, facilitators will encounter children who say that they have not done anything nice for anyone this week. Or children may remark that no one has done anything positive for them over the past few days. Facilitators have an important task here and that is to help children understand once again, that positive interpersonal encounters can occur anytime and anywhere, and that these acts do not have to be huge to earn the label of "kindness". Sharing a smile, thanking a teacher and giving a compliment are all small gestures that children can do at home, in school and around their neighbourhood that would gradually increase children's repertoire of positive behaviours. If children still fail to come up with examples of deeds of kindness after further explanation and prompting, the facilitator could ask children to relate a random day's events (e.g., "Keng Lee, can you tell me how yesterday was like for you? What did you do that was particularly fun and interesting? Did you go anywhere with your parents or friends?"). Typically, from the child's narration of the day's events and encounters, the facilitator would then be able to select certain positive acts that took place and use these as examples of acts of kindness.

2. *Effective Problem-Solving*

- Problem-solving training involves teaching children to think in a goal-directed fashion before acting. Through this type of training, children learn to recognise problems, generate alternative strategies, think of the consequences associated to each proposed solution, anticipate possible obstacles and implement effective strategies to solve social problems. Children of all ages can benefit from problem-solving training in varying degrees. However, parents, teachers and counsellors should note that children eight years and above are more able to apply these strategies to their own problems.

- The five steps in effective problem-solving are:
  1. (Feeling) **A**ngry?
  2. **N**ot to React First
  3. **G**enerate Solutions
  4. **E**valuate Solutions
  5. **R**eflect and reward — Did It Work?

- Rather than just reading these steps for the children, it is generally more educational for the facilitator to encourage the children to generate ideas about what these steps might be, and guide them towards coming up with the five steps.

- **Step 1: (Feeling) Angry?**
  — The first step towards problem-solving is to recognise that there is a problem. Who or what caused the problem? And most importantly, is the person feeling angry about the problem? If not, the subsequent steps are pointless.

— Example: In school, a peer is teasing me and calling me names. I feel quite angry about it.

■ **Step 2: Not to React First**

— Teach the children to stop and not react first. To illustrate this point, ask the children to imagine themselves to be frozen in the moment or to "freeze" or "pause" like a song on their music player. During this moment, they can then be encouraged to think about what they want to achieve. Children can state more than one goal.

— This step is generally less intuitive and more difficult for children to generate on their own, independently.

Examples: a) I want him to stop teasing me.

b) I want to be safe.

c) I don't want to look cowardly or look like a wimp.

d) I don't want to get into trouble.

■ **Step 3: Generate Solutions**

— Children with behavioural problems are less able to generate alternatives to aggression. They often limit their options to the use of physical and/or verbal aggression.

— Examples: a) I could talk to him assertively and say something to him and hopefully get him to stop bothering me.

b) I could threaten him back and beat him up.

c) I could ignore him.

— Allow children to generate multiple possible solutions to the problem. Some solutions generated may be negative and antisocial, and this is permissible and should be allowed. In fact, it is important that children offer unwise and aggressive solutions (e.g., I could beat the person up) so that these solutions can be evaluated at Step 4 just like the other proposed solutions. The evaluation process in Step 4 will allow children to see why certain proposed solutions are not viable or will not meet their goals. If children are prevented from suggesting antisocial solutions at this stage, one of two things might happen. First, they could feel that this problem-solving model is a farce and might subsequently pay lip service to facilitators by giving all the socially appropriate answers but learn nothing through the process. Second, if these antisocial solutions are eliminated at Step 3, this will not allow the facilitator the educational opportunity to evaluate these solutions and explain to the children the reasons why certain solutions are not viable.

▪ Step 4: Evaluate Solutions

— The solutions proposed in the previous step are considered in terms of their likely consequences. This is an important step as it is generally the one that children skip when they deal with conflict. Consequences should be considered in relation to goals specified in Step 2. Children should ask themselves this question, "If I try this solution, will I be meeting most of my goals?"

— Examples: a) If I ignore him, he may not stop. I'll look as if I'm a coward but I will be safe and I won't get into trouble.

b) If I say something to him, he might stop. I won't look as if I'm a coward, I won't get into trouble, and I will be safe (depending on how I say it).

c) If I retaliate aggressively, he might stop. I won't look as if I'm a coward, I will get into trouble and I will not be safe.

— Solution (c) will likely result in the failure to meet two very important goals.

— In addition, consequences should be considered in relation to the application of empathy and perspective-taking skills. Draw on concepts learnt in Session 5.

— Guide the children to make a decision about which solution to implement based on the consideration of its likely consequences and likely fulfilment of specified goals. Based on the examples provided in step 4, being assertive to the teaser seems like an appropriate solution. The facilitator can discuss with the children what types of assertive statements could be used to solve the problem. Facilitators can also stress to the children that ignoring the teaser could be another possible solution depending on the circumstances. Most problems can be resolved with more than one good solution.

— Following that, the decision is then implemented. This is the active step in the ANGER Plan. This portion of Step 4 is more difficult than it appears. Thinking of a good plan or solution does not mean that the child can actually carry out the plan. Children may need to consider external resources such as seeking help from parents or teachers in carrying out the plan.

— For both Steps 4, 5, if the children have difficulty comprehending the terms 'generate' and 'evaluate', the facilitator can use alternative words and phrases such as 'to come up with' and 'compare' respectively, in order to increase understanding.

- **Step 5: Reflect and Reward — Did It Work?**

  — After the problem-solving attempt has been made, it is important to look back on the decision and evaluate whether or not the choice was a good one.

  — If the decision was not a good one, consider other alternatives that can be attempted. Draw on skills learnt in Sessions 3 to 8.

- Figure 2 shows the summary of the ANGER Plan.

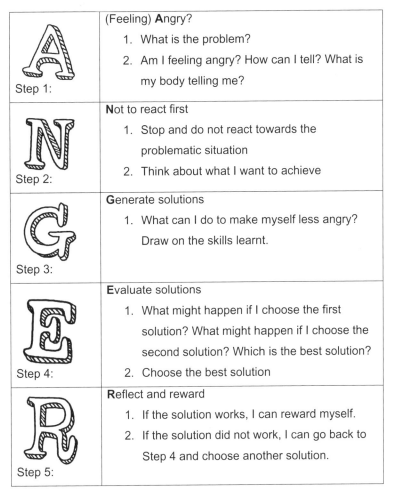

A Step 1:	**(Feeling) A**ngry? 1. What is the problem? 2. Am I feeling angry? How can I tell? What is my body telling me?
N Step 2:	**N**ot to react first 1. Stop and do not react towards the problematic situation 2. Think about what I want to achieve
G Step 3:	**G**enerate solutions 1. What can I do to make myself less angry? Draw on the skills learnt.
E Step 4:	**E**valuate solutions 1. What might happen if I choose the first solution? What might happen if I choose the second solution? Which is the best solution? 2. Choose the best solution
R Step 5:	**R**eflect and reward 1. If the solution works, I can reward myself. 2. If the solution did not work, I can go back to Step 4 and choose another solution.

Figure 2.   The ANGER Plan

- After the ANGER Plan has been taught, the facilitator can consider using a quiz to reinforce the concepts learnt. The facilitator can decide on the structure of the quiz and scoring system that would best appeal to the specific group. Examples of the questions include:

a)   What is the ANGER Plan?

b)   Name two ways where you can tell that you are feeling angry when you are at Step 1 (Feeling Angry) of the ANGER plan.

c)   Name Step 2 of the ANGER Plan.

d)   Name the 'ANGER' step that comes after "Not to React First".

e) Describe what you need to do in Step 4 (Evaluate Solutions) of the ANGER Plan.

f) Describe what you should do in the last step (Reflect and Reward) of the ANGER Plan.

3. *Summary*

▪ The facilitator concludes the session with a summary of what the children learnt in the ANGER Plan. It is important to emphasise to children that the ANGER Plan has its limits. Some problems cannot be solved just be applying the ANGER Plan, as it does not control the behaviour of others.

▪ *Homework: ANGER Plan*

As their homework assignment, the facilitator will ask the children to learn and be familiar with the ANGER Plan using "The five-Step ANGER Plan" worksheet.

Session 10: Application of the ANGER Plan I

> *Overview of Activities:*
>
> 1. Review of Session 9 and homework
> 2. Application of the ANGER plan
> 3. Summary

1. *WELCOME* the group.

2. *REVIEW OF SESSION 9 AND HOMEWORK.*

3. *APPLICATION OF THE ANGER PLAN I.* Begin by providing examples of problematic situations. Guide the group in applying the five steps of the ANGER Plan to solve such situations.

4. *HOMEWORK.* Encourage the group to learn the five steps of the ANGER Plan as part of their homework.

5. *CONCLUSION.* Conclude the session by telling the group that the ANGER Plan can be used to solve real-life problems systematically. Finally, tell the group that they will be learning about the application of the ANGER Plan to solve their own problematic situations next week.

Session 10
Application of the ANGER Plan I

1. *Review of Session 9 and Homework*

   ■ The facilitator reviews what was learnt in Session 9 by discussing the homework assignment. In particular, it is helpful to review the five steps of the ANGER Plan using the "ANGER Plan Review" worksheet. Ask participants to share which steps they found particularly difficult. The facilitator can also ask participants to share some of the other problem-solving strategies they utilised.

2. *Application of the ANGER Plan I*

   ■ The focus of this segment is to teach children how to use the ANGER Plan to solve problematic situations. The facilitator can begin by providing examples of problematic situations that are relevant to the children. The facilitator should not attempt to solve problems for the children. Instead, act as a coach and guide the child to help him/her problem-solve on his/her own. Guide the children through the ANGER Plan using either open-ended or forced-choice questions.

   ■ Examples of open-ended questions include the following:

      – "What can you do?"

      – "I'm rather confused. Can you explain it to me? How could you solve that problem?"

      – "What's the first step? What do you do? OK, now what's the next step?"

   ■ Examples of forced-choice questions include the following:

      ■ "You could try [Solution A] or [Solution B]. What do you think might work best?"

- "Well, it looks like you have three options: choosing to do [Solution A], [Solution B], or [Solution C]. Which of the three alternatives do you think would work best for you?"

- Use the "Applying the ANGER Plan" worksheet for children to practice solving real-life problems using the ANGER Plan.

3. *Summary*

- The facilitator concludes the session with a summary of what the children learnt about the application of the ANGER Plan.

- *Homework*: *ANGER Plan*

  As their homework assignment, the facilitator will ask the children to practise the ANGER Plan using the "Applying the ANGER Plan" worksheet.

Session 11: Application of the ANGER Plan II

Overview of Activities:

1. Review of Session 10 and homework
2. Application of the ANGER Plan II
3. Summary

1. *WELCOME* the group.

2. *REVIEW OF SESSION 10 AND HOMEWORK.*

3. *APPLICATION OF THE ANGER PLAN II.* Begin by asking the group to provide examples of the problematic situations they have encountered. Guide the group to apply the five steps of the ANGER Plan in solving such problematic situations.

4. *HOMEWORK.* Encourage the group to use the five steps of the ANGER Plan to solve their problems as part of their homework.

5. *CONCLUSION.* Conclude the session by telling the group that the ANGER Plan can be used to solve problems systematically. Finally, tell the group that the following meeting will be their final session.

Session 11
Application of the ANGER Plan II

1. *Review of Session 10 and Homework*

   ▪ The facilitator reviews what was learnt in Session 10 by discussing the homework assignment. Ask the children to share which steps they found particularly difficult. Review the five steps of the ANGER Plan if necessary (see "ANGER Plan Review" worksheet from Session 10).

2. *Application of the ANGER Plan II*

   ▪ The focus of this segment is to teach children how to solve their own problems using the ANGER Plan. The facilitator will explore and process with the participants the situations they encountered this week. Ask the children to come up with problematic situations they might currently be facing and facilitators can guide them through the problem-solving process. Examples of problematic situations discussed in Session 2 can also be used (see examples identified using the Feeling-Meter).

   ▪ Once the children have identified their problematic situations, use the "Using the ANGER Plan to Resolve My Problem" worksheet to get them to practise solving these problems using the ANGER Plan. Begin with the easier situations (e.g., problems that made the children a little angry) and gradually work towards the more problematic situations (e.g., problems that made the children very angry). Facilitators should not attempt to solve problems for the children. Instead, act as a coach and guide the child to help him/her problem solve on his/her own. Essentially, the role of the facilitator is to respond to children's ongoing problems and dilemmas by guiding them to solve their own problems. Facilitators can guide children through the use of either open-ended or forced-choice questions (see Session 10 for examples of questions).

- Also the facilitators can use this session as a chance to instil to the children that it takes a lot of practice before they can be good at applying the ANGER Plan in the problematic situations they encounter. They can liken the process to learning how to play a musical instrument or learning multiplication tables. It is difficult and foreign at the beginning, but they will get better as they practise more.

3. *Summary*

- The facilitator concludes the session with a summary of what the children learnt about the application of the ANGER Plan in solving their problems.

- *Homework: ANGER Plan*

  As their homework assignment, ask the children to practise solving their problems using the ANGER Plan. The "Using the ANGER Plan to Resolve My Problem" worksheet can be used.

Session 12: Putting It All Together

> *Overview of Activities:*
>
> 1. Review of Session 11 and homework
> 2. Activities for Putting It All Together session
> 3. Empowerment and maintenance of behavioural improvement
> 4. Conclusion

1. *WELCOME* the group.

2. *REVIEW OF SESSION 11 AND HOMEWORK.*

3. *ACTIVITIES FOR THE PUTTING IT ALL TOGETHER SESSION.* Have the group participate in the activity using the materials provided in Appendix 10 or Appendix 11. This activity would require the group to apply the lessons learnt regarding identification of feelings, anger-coping techniques, empathy, perspective-taking, fighting fair, building prosocial skills and the ANGER Plan.

4. *EMPOWERMENT AND MAINTENANCE OF BEHAVIOURAL IMPROVEMENT.* Encourage and foster the belief that group members have the capacity to cope with problematic situations because they have learnt various coping skills. Remind them to set realistic and manageable goals for themselves as they strive to improve their behaviour.

5. *CONCLUSION.*

Session 12
Putting It All Together

1. *Review of Session 11 and Homework*

   ■ The facilitator reviews what was learnt in Session 11 by reviewing the homework assignment. Ask the children to share which steps they found particularly difficult when they attempted to solve their problems using the ANGER Plan. Also, discuss whether some of them encountered certain types of problems which went beyond the scope of the five steps of the ANGER Plan and required additional intervention from adults. The facilitator can also ask the participants to share some of the other problem-solving strategies they utilised.

2. *Activities for the Putting It All Together Session*

   ■ The facilitator can have group members participate in one or more of the following suggested activities:

   a) Review of Concepts Learnt

   ■ The facilitator can also use an alternative activity called the "The Strongest Link", which is adapted from a UK television game show, to help the children to revise all the concepts learnt. The facilitator can divide the children into two groups and have them compete against each

Levels	Points
1	50
2	100
3	150
4	200
5	300
6	400
7	500
8	600

other. The idea is to have one group of children taking turns to answer questions relating to the entire programme. The goal is for the team to answer eight questions correctly in a consecutive manner to earn the maximum points (50 + 100 + 150....+ 600 = 2300 points) for their team (see scoring table on the right). If an incorrect answer is given, the points they have accumulated thus far will be forfeited entirely. The next question will be only worth the first level of points (i.e., 50 points). The game will stop when the team has finished answering all eight questions and the facilitator will move onto the next team. The facilitator can decide on the rules of the activity. An example list of questions is included in Appendix 10.

b) *Understanding the Human Experience Through Sharing*

■ This activity is designed to have children demonstrate the skills they have acquired thus far and serves as an integrative summary of the 12-session problem-solving, social skills programme. This activity requires participants to demonstrate respect for others by displaying adequate skills in listening, sharing and respectful communication. The activity cards are provided in Appendix 11. The facilitator can choose to use all the cards or use only certain cards depending on the number and composition of group members. It is hoped that children will apply the lessons learnt regarding identification of feelings, anger-coping techniques, empathy, perspective-taking, fighting fair, prosocial skills and the ANGER Plan as they participate in this final activity.

■ Children participating in the group take turns to draw a card and respond to it while the facilitator moderates the discussion, ensuring that individuals do not interrupt others, say something to hurt the feelings of another person or do something to provoke another person. If this activity is used as a classroom activity for approximately 40 pupils, the teacher can divide the class into five groups with each group consisting of eight pupils. The same set of activity cards can be used for each sub-group of eight pupils. The teacher moves from group to group within the classroom facilitating the process and helping with group discussions. If facilitators are working with individual children, it will be a good idea to take turns in responding to these activity cards with the child. This way, the child would not feel as if he/she is sitting for an oral examination. In addition, the facilitator's sharing of personal information through participation in the activity encourages the child to do likewise.

- Because the nature of this activity requires children to discuss or share thoughts and feelings on more personal and/or sensitive issues, it is of paramount importance that facilitators stay vigilant and prevent any kind of name-calling among group members. In order to conduct this activity successfully with the children fully invested and engaged in the process, put-downs, teasing, name-calling or any other form of disrespectful behaviour should not be tolerated. Sharing at a more intimate level such as this requires all participants to respect individual, familial, cultural and religious differences among participants.

3. *Empowerment*

- Another critical component of the last intervention session is empowerment. The facilitator needs to empower children by encouraging and believing that they have the capacity to gradually overcome these various behavioural difficulties on their own. Novice facilitators may sometimes mistakenly assume that children will hold them in higher esteem if they appear to be expert users of this powerful intervention programme that somehow magically solves complex behavioural problems. In fact, effective facilitators are ones who demystify the intervention process and explain to participants that there is little that is mysterious or magical about the intervention. On the contrary, for the programme to work, it requires consistency, hard work and practice on the part of each participant. It is one thing to learn various skills, strategies and approaches to positive coping and problem-solving, but quite another thing to consistently and conscientiously apply these principles in our lives when we are caught in unpleasant situations or when we are interacting with difficult people. Empower children by encouraging them to continue to apply what they have learnt in their daily interactions with other people. When children feel empowered, their self-esteem is raised and consequently, they will gradually learn to take responsibility for their behaviour.

- An example of an activity that can be a platform to empower the children is "Me: Before and After".

The facilitator can provide the children with two pieces of coloured paper and some art medium. Ask the children to draw a picture of how they were like before the start of Session 1, and how they are like right now (Session 12). The idea is to keep the instruction as open-ended as possible for the children to make their own reflection about how the sessions have helped (or not helped) them. After all the children have completed their drawings, the facilitator can have the children share and elaborate what they have drawn. Examples of questions for discussion: How do they deal with angry situations differently now? What has changed in them? What is the biggest learning point from the sessions? Here, the children have the opportunity to see for themselves and come up with their own observation on the changes.

- The facilitators should also be mindful that there might be a small handful of children who might be reluctant to indicate what improvements they have made. In such cases, the facilitators can help the children to identify at least one positive change and encourage them to continue working on it to maximise gains.

4. *Maintenance of Behavioural Improvement*

- There are two important points for children to remember: a) improvement in behaviour is a gradual process, and b) setbacks are not necessarily failures.

- Facilitators need to emphasise to participants that improvement in behaviour can be a long, slow and tedious process. Thus, it is crucial that participants set realistic and manageable goals for themselves as they strive to improve their behaviour. Break the goal down into small, bite-sized steps. Negative behaviour patterns or habits take time to develop. Anyone attempting to get rid of a bad habit will recognise that established habits are not easy to break. In addition, this programme hopes to not only reduce negative behaviour patterns, but also to increase positive behaviour patterns. It is also helpful for participants to remember that setbacks are normal and to be expected.

There will be many times in which participants will encounter setbacks, but these should not be interpreted as failures. Rather, setbacks can be viewed as learning experiences and opportunities for further growth and development.

5. *Conclusion*

- Get each child to write some words of encouragement for each other.

- Some facilitators may choose to conduct a couple of "booster" sessions three or six months after the completion of the intervention programme. The purpose of these "booster" sessions is to remind participants of what was previously learnt and to re-teach some lessons that may have been forgotten. Sometimes, conducting these "booster" sessions may not be feasible. For example, some students who participated in the intervention programme may have been graduating students (e.g., Primary 6) who may no longer be in the school three or six months post-intervention. While it is helpful to conduct a couple of "booster" sessions for the children, it may not always be feasible. If facilitators decide to conduct "booster" sessions, they may choose to conduct either one or two "booster" sessions. They can decide to schedule two "booster" sessions one week apart from each other or they can choose to conduct one "booster" session three months post-intervention and another "booster" session six months post-intervention.

- Finally, the importance of the facilitator's role cannot be overemphasised. As the teacher, counsellor or parent facilitates the intervention programme, he/she is constantly modelling appropriate behaviour and attitudes. As the saying goes, "Values are better caught than taught". Sometimes, the most important lesson you teach the children is communicated by the way you behave, rather than by what you say.

Appendix 1
Friendship Bingo Blank Template

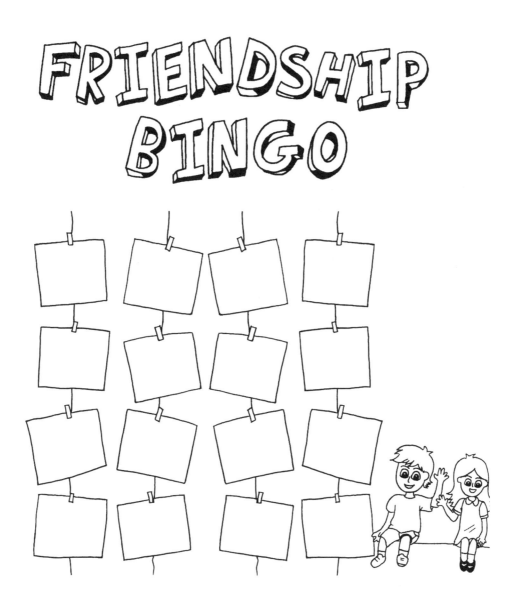

Appendix 2
Feeling Cards

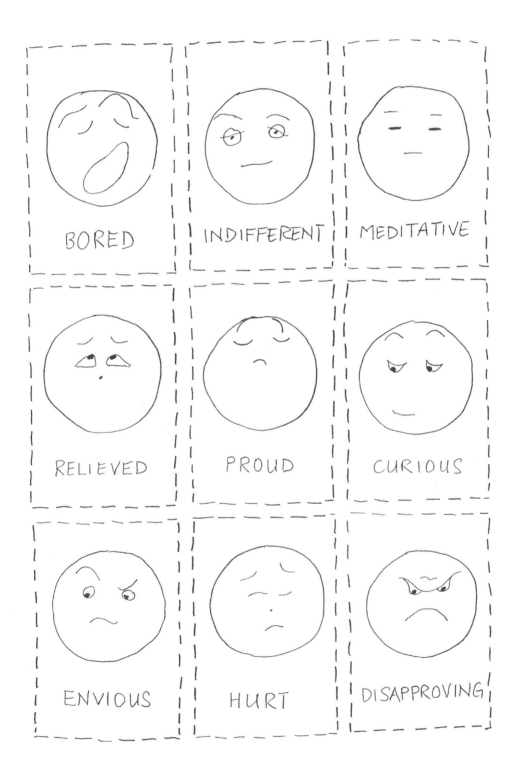

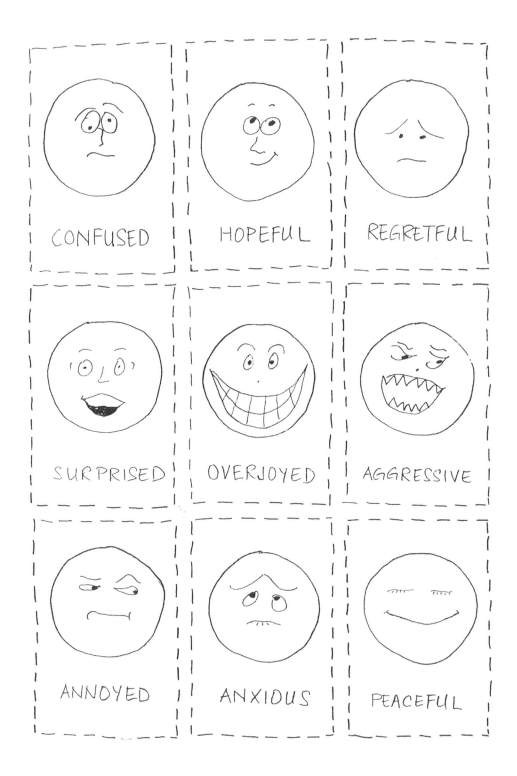

CONFUSED   HOPEFUL   REGRETFUL

SURPRISED   OVERJOYED   AGGRESSIVE

ANNOYED   ANXIOUS   PEACEFUL

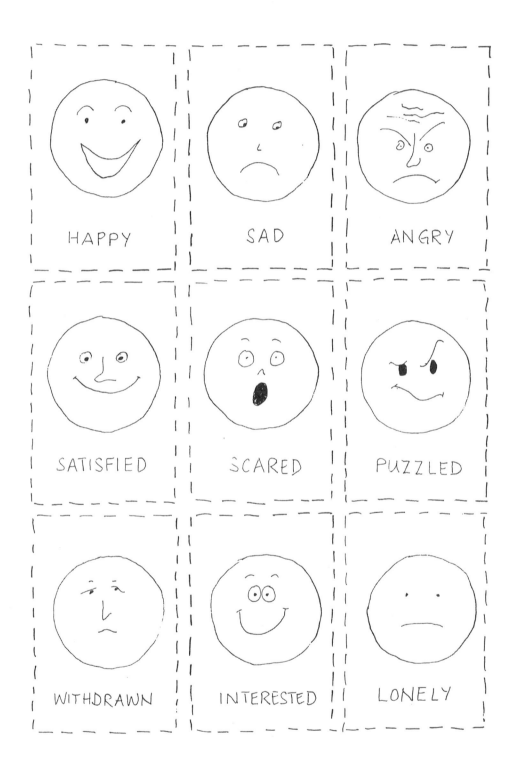

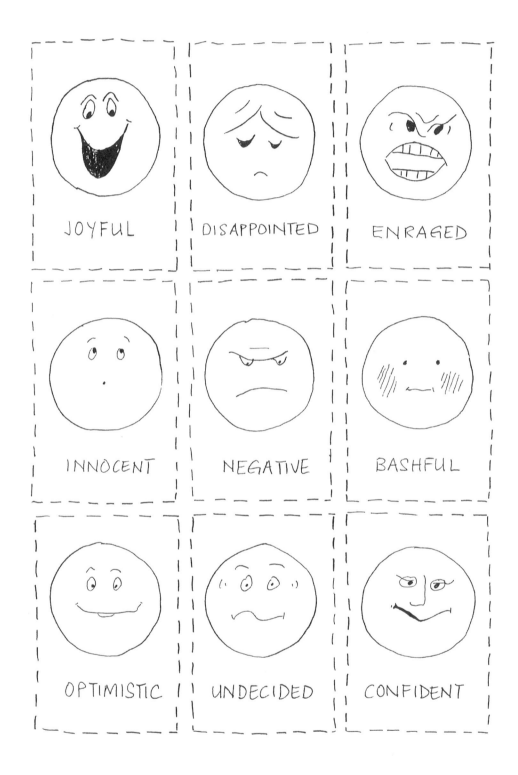

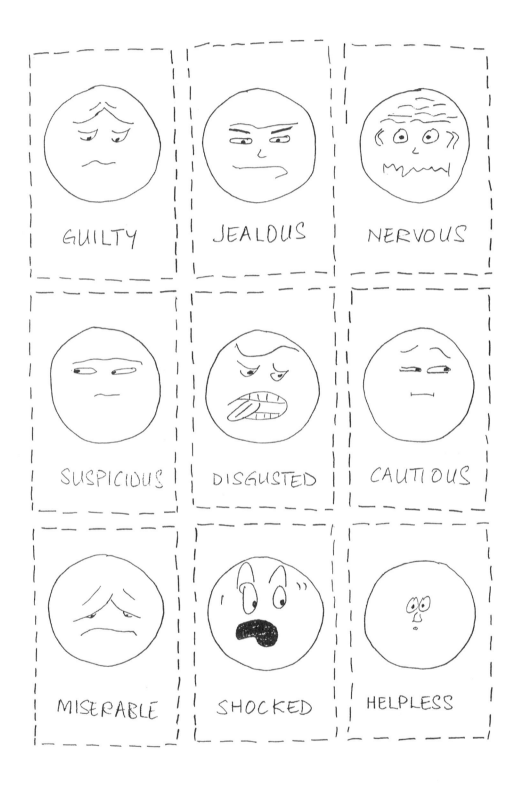

Appendix 3
Feelings Word Bank

Here is a list of <u>Pleasant</u> and <u>Unpleasant</u> feeling words that you might have come across or experienced before. You may add more of your own!

PLEASANT

Joy/Happiness
Delighted
Glad
Sunny
Cheerful
Gleeful
Joyful
Excited
Jolly
Grateful
Wonderful
Lighthearted
Zest
Elated
Optimistic
Amused
_____
_____
_____
_____

Love
Loved
Affectionate
Considerate
Touched
Sympathy
Comforted
Warmth
Tender
Understanding
Friendly
Admired
Devoted
_____
_____
_____
_____

Positive
Eager
Keen
Determined
Enthusiastic
Confident
Free & Easy
Energetic
Wonderful
Courageous
Encouraged
_____
_____
_____
_____

UNPLEASANT

Anger
Annoyed
Irritated
Upset
Mean
Grumpy
Frustrated
Mad
Cross
Impatient
Insulted
Enraged
_____
_____
_____
_____

Sadness
Unhappy
Gloomy
Hopeless
Tearful
Discouraged
Lonely
Disappointed
Dismayed
Pained
Grieved
Desperate
Pessimistic
_____
_____
_____
_____

Fear
Anxious
Panic
Scared
Nervous
Timid
Frightened
Alarmed
Suspicious
Terrified
Shock
Dread
Tense
_____
_____
_____
_____

Appendix 4
Scripts for Breathing Exercises, Visualisation and Tense-and-Relax

Breathing Exercises

Step 1:

- Sit comfortably on a chair. Put your hands on your lap.

- Focus your attention on your breathing.

Step 2:

- Close your eyes.

- Breathe in slowly through your nose (put your hand on your belly to feel it rise).

- Hold your breath (count 1 to 4).

Step 3:

- Breathe out slowly through your mouth (put your hand on your belly to feel it sink).

Step 4:

Repeat Steps 1 to 3 for as many times as you wish.

Visualisation and Deep Breathing Exercises

Step 1:

- Sit comfortably on a chair. Put your hands on your lap.

- Focus your attention on your breathing.

Step 2:

- Close your eyes.

- Breathe in slowly through your nose (put your hand on your belly to feel it rise).

- Hold your breath (count 1 to 4).

Step 3:

- Breathe out slowly through your mouth (put your hand on your belly to feel it sink).

Step 4:

While doing these breathing exercises, use your imagination to fill your mind with calm, relaxing pictures such as beautiful natural scenes. You may also think of calming words such as 'relax'.

Step 5:

Repeat Steps 1 to 4 for as many times as you wish.

Tense-and-Relax

Step 1: Let's begin to relax the muscles in your body starting from your face. Pretend you are an old man or woman and squeeze your nose to make as many wrinkles on your face as possible. Squeeze as hard as you can. Hold for five counts. Slowly let go and relax. Now, close your eyes as tightly as you can. Hold for five counts. Open your eyes slowly and relax.

Step 2: Now, let's work on your jaw muscles. Pretend that you have a hard piece of candy in your mouth and try to bite through it. Bite hard. Hold for five counts. Slowly let go of the candy.

Step 3: Now, let's work on your shoulders. Pretend that you are carrying a heavy schoolbag. Try to lift the schoolbag as high as you can with your shoulders. Lift as high as you can. Hold for five counts. Slowly release your shoulders.

Now, pretend that you have a ball in your right hand and squeeze as hard as you can. Hold for five counts. Now, let go of the ball and relax. (Repeat for the left hand.)

Step 4: Let's work on your legs now starting with your right leg. Lift your right leg slightly above the ground and point your toes to the ground without touching it. Hold for five counts. Relax and now, point your toes to the sky. Again, hold for five counts and relax. (Repeat for the left leg.)

Step 5: Now you have learnt the ways to tense and relax your muscles. Whenever you feel angry, take a few minutes to tighten your muscles then relax them. Feel the tension in your body go away.

Note:

1. It is a good idea to begin with some breathing exercises prior to practicing the tense-and-relax strategy.

2. For each step, repeat as many times as needed.

3. Modify the script according to the needs of your group.

Appendix 5
Story-telling Techniques: Word Cue Cards

"bad"

"wound"

"hit"

"punch"

"argue"

"cry"

"lost the game"

"forgot to bring his/her Maths textbook"

"failed the final exam"

"not playing attention"

"daydreaming"

"slipped and fell"

"cheating"

"teased him/her"

"called him/her 'fatso'"

"came in last for the competition"

"frustrated"

"angry"

"hate"

"stare"

"gang fight"

"grumbling"

"bleeding profusely"

"his/her plans failed"

Appendix 6
Vignettes and Instructions

Instructions:

I am going to read you a short vignette or story about things that happen to children. I will also show you some pictures to help you see what is happening in the story. I will also ask you some questions about the stories.

Vignette 1

You are about to climb up the monkey bars. You see two boys playing with a ball nearby. Just as you swing across the bars, you get hit hard in the back with the ball that was thrown by the boy nearby.

Discussion Questions for Vignette 1

1) What do you think happened? If the child does not spontaneously generate an intent, ask: Why do you think he hit you with the ball?

2) I'm going to describe two scenarios. I want you to tell me in which scenario would it be more likely that the boy deliberately hit you with the ball. The first scenario is when the two boys are playing very far away from the monkey bars and the ball hits you. The second scenario is when the two boys are playing nearby and the ball hits you. If both scenarios happened to you, in which of the scenarios do you think it might have been accidental and in which of the scenarios do you think it might have been deliberate?

3) Let's pretend that the boy who threw the ball that hit you wore thick glasses and cannot see very well. In this case, do you think it was done on purpose or was it an accident?

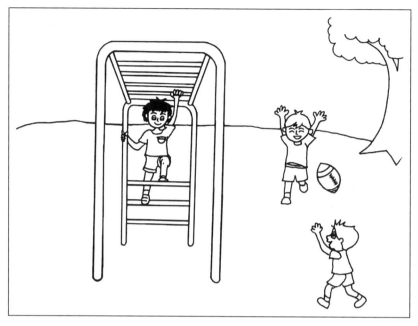

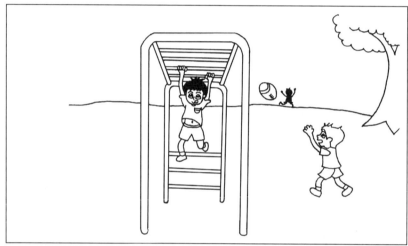

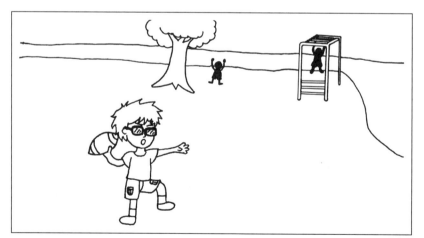

Vignette 2

It's recess time and you just bought a bowl of laksa and a glass of coca cola after being in the queue for a long time. Suddenly, you get knocked on the back and your tray together with your laksa and coca cola spills all over the floor. When you turn around, you see that a girl has knocked into you with her tray.

Discussion Questions for Vignette 2

1) What do you think happened? If the child does not spontaneously generate an intent, ask: Why do you think she knocked you?

2) I'm going to describe two scenarios. I want you to tell me in which scenario would it be more likely that the girl deliberately knocked you. The first scenario is when the canteen is very crowded and the girl knocks into you. The second scenario is when the canteen is quite empty and the girl knocks into you. If both scenarios happened to you, in which of the scenarios do you think it might have been accidental and in which of the scenarios do you think it might have been deliberate?

3) Let's pretend that the girl that knocked into you stepped onto a patch of oil that was on the canteen floor. In this case, do you think it was done on purpose or was it an accident?

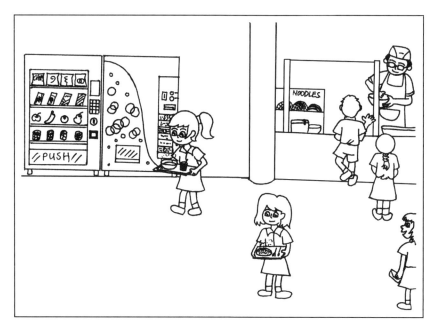

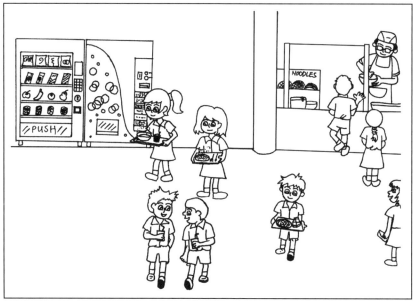

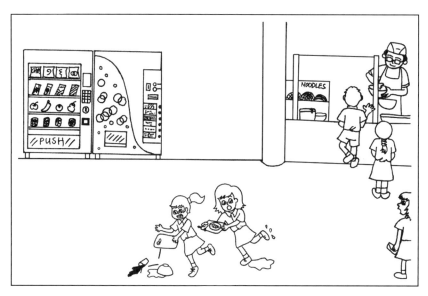

Vignette 3

You are walking along the pavement after school. It rained earlier in the afternoon and there are many mud puddles on the road. You see a boy riding by on his bicycle. As he rides by you, he hits a puddle and mud splashes all over you.

Discussion Questions for Vignette 3

1) What do you think happened? If the child does not spontaneously generate an intent, ask: Why do you think he splashed mud on you?

2) I'm going to describe two scenarios. I want you to tell me in which scenario would it be more likely that the boy deliberately splashed mud on you. The first scenario is when there is a bus also moving in the same left lane as the cyclist, and the road is fairly congested. The second scenario is when the road is completely clear and free of traffic except for the cyclist. If both scenarios happened to you, in which of the scenarios do you think it might have been accidental and in which of the scenarios do you think it might have been deliberate?

3) Let's pretend that the cyclist that splashed mud on you learnt to ride a bicycle not too long ago and is still not very good with balancing himself on the bicycle. In this case, do you think it was done on purpose or was it an accident?

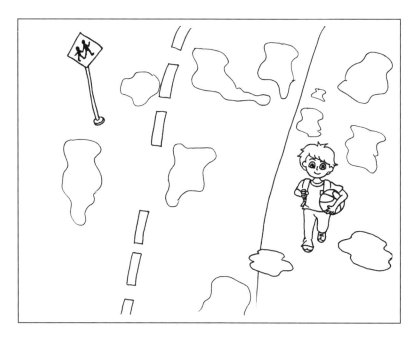

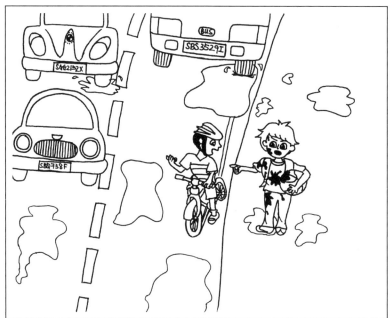

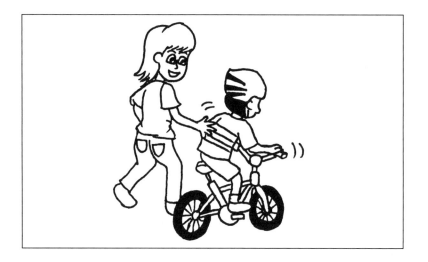

Vignette 4

You have just finished Art class. You have built your model house and left it on your desk for the paint to dry and the glue to set. A girl walks by and as she makes her way towards the teacher's desk, she knocks into your desk. Your model falls off and breaks into pieces.

Discussion Questions for Vignette 4

1) What do you think happened? If the child does not spontaneously generate an intent, ask: Why do you think she knocked into your desk?

2) I'm going to describe two scenarios. I want you to tell me in which scenario would it be more likely that girl deliberately knocked into you. The first scenario is when there are lots of pupils walking around in the classroom because Art class has just ended and everyone is either keeping their materials or going to the washroom to wash their hands. The second scenario is when all pupils are in their seats except for this one girl who needed to see the teacher. If both scenarios happened to you, in which of the scenarios do you think it might have been accidental and in which of the scenarios do you think it might have been deliberate?

3) Let's pretend that the girl that knocked into your desk has recently fractured her leg. Her leg is still in a cast and she is currently using crutches to help her to walk. In this case, do you think it was done on purpose or was it an accident?

Vignette 5

You represented your school in a basketball tournament. During the game, one of the members from the opposing team tried to snatch the ball from you and made you fall.

Discussion Questions for Vignette 5

1) What do you think happened? If the child does not spontaneously generate an intent, ask: Why do you think he/she made you fall?

2) I'm going to describe two scenarios. I want you to tell me in which scenario would it be more likely that he/she deliberately knocked onto you and made you fall. The first scenario is he/she lost his/her balance when he/she was trying to snatch the ball from you. The second scenario is when he/she elbowed you in the stomach while trying to snatch the ball. If both scenarios happened to you, in which of the scenarios do you think it might have been accidental and in which of the scenarios do you think it might have been deliberate?

3) Let's pretend that he/she lost his/her balance while trying to snatch the ball from you. In this case, do you think it was done on purpose or was it an accident?

Vignette 6

You are walking towards your seat after talking to the teacher. On your way, you trip and fall. When you turn around, you see the boy who tripped you with his leg.

Discussion Questions for Vignette 6

1) What do you think happened? If the child does not spontaneously generate an intent, ask: Why do you think the boy tripped you?

2) I'm going to describe two scenarios. I want you to tell me in which scenario would it be more likely that he deliberately tripped you. The first scenario is when the boy saw you coming and he puts his leg out to block your way. The second scenario is when the boy dropped his pen and bent down to pick it up without noticing you coming. If both scenarios happened to you, in which of the scenarios do you think it might have been accidental and in which of the scenarios do you think it might have been deliberate?

3) Let's pretend that the boy dropped his pen and bent down to pick it up. In this case, do you think it was done on purpose or was it an accident?

Appendix 7
Fighting Fair Role-Playing Cards

Both Amran and Nona wanted their mother to help them with homework at the same time. What would be a good solution to this problem? What would have to happen for it to work?

Kok Chuan and Benjamin are classmates and they usually enjoy playing sports or board games together. During recess earlier today, Kok Chuan wanted to play in the school field, while Benjamin wanted to stay indoors. How can Kok Chuan and Benjamin each do what they wanted without fighting?

Ai-Leen called Nalini "a stupid fool" when Nalini accidentally tore Ai-Leen's new book. Nalini thought, "I'm not stupid. It was just an accident." How might Ai-Leen and Nalini resolve this problem with a win-win solution?

Osman kicked the soccer ball right into Teck Wai's stomach. Teck Wai thought, "I feel like kicking the ball right at his face!" How might Osman and Teck Wai resolve this problem in an appropriate manner?

Meiling and Limei were asked by their parents to help them run the drinks stall for one day. They could keep the day's profits as extra pocket money. Meiling thought that she deserved more money when they divided up their profits because she worked harder. Limei felt this is unfair. Come up with a win-win solution.

Mohan and Rafi do not get along with each other. Mohan is better than Rafi in Maths but does not help Rafi out when Rafi gets stuck on a Maths problem even when Rafi approaches him for help. Rafi recently got a pair of new rollerblades for Christmas. He began to make fun of Mohan's old and worn-out rollerblades and even got several other classmates to gang up against Mohan calling him nasty names. Mohan was both upset and angry. How can they get along better? Come up with a win-win solution.

Li Rong called Sharifyah a "stupid kiasu jerk" because Sharifyah wouldn't let Li Rong copy her English homework. How will Li Rong and Sharifyah resolve this conflict? Come up with a good solution.

Prasad kept staring at Aziz throughout lunch. Prasad thought, "If he doesn't stop staring at me, I'm going to beat him up." What can Prasad and Aziz do to handle this situation in an appropriate way?

Appendix 8
Activity Cards: Teaching Prosocial Skills

What would you do if your friends had a packet of sweets that you wanted him to share with you?

What would you do if your classmate was hogging the computer and you wanted to use it?

Name some ways you can help your mother.

Describe a game in which you have to cooperate in order to win.

During a football game, someone bumped into you and did not apologise. What would you do?

Someone bumped into you in the canteen and made you drop your food. What would you do?

Describe a game in which you have to cooperate in order to win.

What makes a successful team?

If you wanted to play a game but your friends wanted to play something else, what could you do?

If this is the first day in a new class at school, what could you do to make friends?

What would you do if one of your classmate calls you a coward?

What could you do if you see your teacher having some difficulty carrying a pile of books?

In what ways can
you help a friend?

You see a new boy in class.
What could you do
to befriend him?

This is the first day in a new
class at school. How do
you react if someone
comes up to you and
says "Hello"?

The person sitting next to
you in class is having
difficulty understanding
what the teacher says.
What could you do?

What do you say or do
when someone introduces
you to a stranger?

Name some ways you
can show cooperation.

Describe a story from books, TV or movies about teamwork.

Describe two situations where you need to share.

What could you do to form a friendship that lasts?

Name two things that you could do with your friend.

What could your team do to win a basketball match?

What could you do if you and your sister want to watch different TV programmes at the same time?

Name some ways you can show cooperation.

If your brother has already eaten 10 sticks of satay and you had only eaten three, and your mother wanted you to give him the last satay stick, what would you do?

If you were stuck with a Maths problem, who would you approach for help?

Name some ways in which you could help in a Senior Citizens' home.

Name some things that you can share with others.

A friend whom you loaned some money to is now refusing to pay you back. What would you do?

Describe two situations where adults should cooperate more.

How could you and your sister cooperate if both of you needed the computer urgently to finish your homework?

What qualities would make you a good friend to others?

Describe a story from books, TV or movies about friends helping each other.

You see a new boy in class. How do you strike a conversation with him? Role-play the situation.

Why is it important to cooperate in a football game?

How would you react if a new student in class comes up to you and teases you?

What would you do if you found out that someone has been telling tales behind your back?

During a badminton tournament, your partner accidentally hits you with his racket. What would you do?

Why does one need to make friends?

Appendix 9
Questions for "The Strongest Link" Quiz

Identification of Feelings and Exploring Anger Feelings

1. Identify this feeling. [Show a picture]

2. Give two examples of pleasant feelings.

3. Give two examples of unpleasant feelings.

4. List two cues that would enable one to know how a person is feeling at the moment.

5. Anger is a normal feeling that everyone experiences but we can control how we react towards the situation. [True/False]

6. Give two examples of how your body would respond when you are feeling angry.

7. Give two examples of angry thoughts.

8. What is one possible negative consequence if one were to express his/her anger explosively?

9. Name two of the three Anger Rules.

Anger-Coping Techniques I and II

10. Name one activity that you've learnt to calm yourself down when you are irritated or agitated.

11. Demonstrate how to do deep breathing.

12. Demonstrate how to do the tense-and-relax technique.

13. What does 'Fi' in FiSH stand for?

14. How would an assertive person respond to something he/she does not agree to?

15. Demonstrate how you would speak in a FiRM manner.

16. Give two possible sources of social support.

Empathy and Perspective-Taking

17. Empathy means 'walking in another person's shoes'. [True/False]

18. Give an example of how one would demonstrate perspective-taking.

19. Perspective taking means trying to understand another person's point of view. [True/False]

Fighting Fair

20. It is possible for two persons to have separate opinions and they are both right. [True/False]

21. What is CRAWL formula used for?

22. What does the 'L' in CRAWL stand for?

23. Demonstrate what you would do to show that you are taking responsibility for your own action.

24. What is an example of a "foul"?

Prosocial Skills

25. Give an example of prosocial behaviour.

26. Name one way you can show prosocial behaviour when working in a group.

ANGER Plan

27. What does the 'A' in the ANGER plan stand for?

28. What does the 'N' in the ANGER plan stand for?

29. What does the 'G' in the ANGER plan stand for?

30. What does the 'E' in the ANGER plan stand for?

31. What does the 'R' in the ANGER plan stand for?

32. [Jack was playing soccer with his classmates during PE class when a boy he didn't like accidentally tripped him over in the midst of chasing the ball. As Jack fell and hurt his knee, he could hear the opposing team scoring a goal. He started to feel his jaw tighten and his fists clenching......] Imagine you are Jack, apply the ANGER plan and generate two possible solutions. Select the strategy of your choice and explain why.

Appendix 10
Activity Cards: Understanding the Human Experience Through Sharing

If you could choose to relive one year of your life, which year would it be, and why?	Talk about something that happened to you that made you feel disappointed.
How do you choose between what's right and what's wrong?	Stress affects all of us in different ways. Talk about how stress affects you.
Talk about something that happened to you that made you feel hurt.	Say two things you like about yourself. Explain why.
What is something that happened to you that made you feel appreciated? Talk about it.	Say two things you don't like about yourself. Explain why.

Geok Poh sometimes feels envious when her friend has something she does not have. What would make you envious? Talk about it.

When Mary is sad, she wants to eat chocolates. What do you do when you feel sad?

Ali does not want to participate in the competition because he hates to lose. Talk about losing.

Talk about something you do well that makes you feel good about yourself.

What bothers you most about other people?

Say something about a bad habit you are trying to quit.

What is something that happened which made you feel guilty?

Kok Meng is in a wheelchair and cannot walk because he lost his legs in a serious accident a few years ago. What are some things you could do with Kok Meng if you were his friend?

Who can you turn to if you were feeling sad?

Talk about one person who has the biggest impact on your life.

Who is your favourite teacher and why?

Talk about something that happened to you that made you feel like giving up.

When Razak had to give a speech in front of the whole school, he felt nervous. When do you feel nervous?

If you could choose to spend a day with anybody in the whole world, who would it be? Why?

Talk about something that happened to you that made you feel left out.

Talk about something that happened to you that made you feel afraid.

Devraj sometimes talks so much that he doesn't listen to other people. Talk about someone who listens when you talk to them.

What is something you want your classmates to remember about you?

When Jason admitted that he was afraid, he learnt that everyone has fears. Talk about one of your fears.

Talk about something that happened to you that made you feel bored.

Talk about something that happened to you that made you feel embarrassed.

Talk about something that happened to you that made you feel frustrated.

When was the last time you felt "boiling mad"? What happened?

How would you feel if everyone forgot your birthday?

Sometimes it's hard for Jack to be honest. Talk about a time when you found it hard to be honest.

Talk about two things you have learnt in life.

Tommy misplaced Vijay's CD. Tommy and Vijay got into a fight. What do you think about fighting?

Talk about a time when you felt unloved.

Talk about a time you felt ashamed.

Talk about a time you felt confident.

Talk about a time you felt confused.

Talk about a time you felt loved.

Talk about a time
you felt inadequate.

If someone wrote a book
about you, what would the
title be? Why?

Share a hope you have
about the future.

When was/is the happiest
day of your life? What
happened on that day?

Name two people who
have helped you in the past.
What did they do?

Is there someone you
would have liked to
know better but the
opportunity has slipped by?
Talk about it.

What is one question you
always wanted to ask but
never dared to?

If you won a prize of
$1000, how would
you spend it?

What are some things you can do to calm yourself down when someone makes you angry?

If you could choose to be someone else, would you? If your answer is "no", why do you choose to remain yourself? If your answer is "yes", who would you like to be?

Do you believe in keeping promises? Why or why not?

Are you an optimist or a pessimist? Would your friends agree?

If you could ask for anything in the world, what would it be? Why?

If some of your friends in school are asking to you do something you know is wrong, what would you do? How would you handle this?

Complete the sentence: Reading aloud in class makes me feel _____.

Which subject do you dislike the most? Why?

What is something you are thankful for? Talk about it.

What is your response when someone cuts in front of you when you are lining up to buy stamps at the post office?

Padma is new student in your class. What can you do to make her feel welcomed?

How would you react when someone knocks into you? How else could you react?

"There is so much to learn — you can never learn enough." Do you agree or disagree? Why?

Some individuals feel that they would be the happiest people in the world if they had lots of money. Is it true? Why or why not?

Say something about competitiveness. Do you feel being competitive is good? Explain.

Don cheered his friend up when his friend was feeling down. Have you ever tried to cheer someone up? Talk about it.

References

Introduction

- Crick, N. R., & Dodge, K. A. (1994). A review and reformulation of social information processing mechanisms in children's social adjustment. Psychological Bulletin, 115, 74–101.
- Meichenbaum, D. (1977). Cognitive-behaviour modification. New York: Plenum Press.
- Shapiro, E. S., & Cole, C. L. (1994). Behaviour change in the classroom: Self-management interventions. New York: Guilford Press.

Session 1

- Dodge, K. A., Laird, R., Lochman, J. E., Zelli, A., & Conduct Problems Prevention Research Group. (2002). Multidimensional latent-construct analysis of children's social information processing patterns: Correlations with aggressive behaviour problems. Psychological Assessment, 14, 60–73.
- Kusche, C., & Greenberg, M. (1994). PATHS: Promoting alternative thinking strategies. SouthDeerfield, MA: Developmental Research Programmes Inc.
- Mostow, A. J., Izard, C. E., Fine, S., & Trentacosta, R. (2002). Modeling emotional, cognitive, and behavioural predictors of peer acceptance. Child Development, 73,1775–1787.

Session 3

- Conrad, A., & Roth, W. (2007). Muscle relaxation therapy for anxiety disorders: It works but how? Journal of Anxiety Disorders, 21, 243–264.
- Dolbier, C. L., & Rush, T. E. (2012). Efficacy of abbreviated progressive muscle relaxation in a high-stress college sample. International Journal of Stress Management, 19, 48–68.
- Kellner, M. H., Bry, B. H., & Salvador, D. S. (2008). Anger management effects on middle school students with emotional/behavioural disorders: Anger log use, aggressive and prosocial behaviour, Child & Family Behaviour Therapy, 30, 215–230.

- Sukhodolsky, D. G., Vitulano, L. A., Carroll, D. H., McGuire, J., Leckman, J. F., & Scahill, L. (2009). Randomised trial of anger control training for adolescents with Tourette's syndrome and disruptive behaviour. Journal of the American Academy of Child and Adolescent Psychiatry, 48, 413–421.
- Weisz, J. R., & Gray, J. S. (2008). Evidence-based psychotherapy for children and adolescents: Data from the present and a model for the future. Child and Adolescent Mental Health, 13, 54–65.

Session 4

- Harris, A. R., & Walton, M. D. (2009). "Thank you for making me write this." Narrative skills and the management of conflict in urban schools. Urban Review, 41, 287–311.
- Nicolopoulou, A. (2007). From actors to agents to persons: The development of character representation in young children's narratives. Child Development, 78(2), 412–429.
- Smith, J. (2009). Blending effective behaviour management and literacy strategies for preschoolers exhibiting negative behaviour. Early Childhood Education Journal, 37, 147–151.

Session 5

- Dadds, M. R., Hawes, D. J., Frost, A. D., Vassallo, V., Bunn, P., Hunter, K., & Merz, S. (2008). The measurement of empathy in children using parent reports. Journal of Child Psychiatry and Human Development, 39, 111–122.
- Eisenberg, N., Spinrad, T. L., & Sadovsky, A. (2006). Empathy-related responding in children. In M. Killen, & J. Smetana (Eds.), Handbook of Moral Development (pp. 517–549). Mahwah, NJ: Erlbaum.
- Hoffman, M. L. (2000). Empathy and moral development: Implications for caring and justice. Cambridge, UK: Cambridge University Press.

Session 6

- Hughes, J. N. (1996). Social Cognitive Assessment Profile-Revised. Unpublished test. (Available from author at Department of Educational Psychology, TAMU 4222, Texas A&M University, College Station, TX 77843–4222).

Session 7

- McKay, M., Rogers, P., & McKay, J. (1989). When anger hurts: Quieting the storm within. Oakland, CA: New Harbinger.

Session 8

- Editors of Conari Press. (2002). Random Acts of Kindness. San Francisco, CA: Author.
- Editor of Conari Press. (2013). Random Acts of Kindness Then and Now. The 20th Anniversary of a Simple Idea that Changes Lives. San Francisco, CA: Author.